Meaning-Making and Wellbeing: Positive Psychology Interventions for Hearing Voices

Seusspie

TABLE OF CONTENTS

CHAPTER I

INTRODUCTION

In Chapter 1, I introduce my topic: clinicians' use of a positive psychology framework with people with psychotic experiences, and experiences of client conceptualization and intervention approaches that exist among practitioners of both counseling and clinical psychology backgrounds. First, I provide a brief overview of how the medical model came to dominate the ways in which presenting mental health issues are classified, treated, and understood. In my historical overview, I provide some background on the emergence of counseling psychology as a field. I then narrow my focus to symptoms of psychosis, including but not limited to people with schizophrenia. I will refer to people who experience psychotic symptoms and meet criteria for a psychotic disorder as people with psychosis but will more frequently reference people who hear voices (including those who do not meet criteria for a psychotic disorder) as healthy voice-hearers or people who hear voices. I discuss some of the challenges that are associated with psychosis and hearing voices, including stigma and psychosocial difficulties. Next, I write about the role of meaning-making in a therapist's work with clients who have psychotic experiences. This content is followed by a discussion on current treatments that are used with people with psychosis, including (a) pharmacologic,

1

(b) Cognitive-Behavioral Therapy (CBT) for psychosis, (c) mindfulness, (d) peer support interventions for psychosis, and (e) treatments for acute psychosis. Next, the discussion shifts to a positive psychology framework, providing an overview of the positive psychology movement and information about positive psychology interventions for psychosis. Finally, a gap in the current literature is introduced; little is presently known about mental health service providers' beliefs about psychosis and hearing voices, as well as how this informs their conceptualization of and clinical work with people with these experiences. This chapter then presents the rationale for the need for research in this area, including the problem statement, the significance of the problem, and the purpose and significance of the proposed study. Finally, implications of this study are discussed; people who hear voices may be better understood by learning about how clinicians view these clients' experiences, and how this research may be used to guide future work.

These implications highlight how this topic is important for increasing understanding of how people experience hearing voices, and how clinicians of all training backgrounds can use evidence-based practice to help clients improve their functioning across multiple areas of life, as well as feel less stigmatized and more understood by mental health providers. Using positive psychology interventions can provide therapists with evidence-based interventions for helping people who hear voices make meaning of their experiences and improve their well-being. Applying a critical theory lens to this work can provide a framework for viewing the experiences of people with psychosis and people who hear voices as marginalized and help to provide tools for advocating and working effectively with these clients.

Historical Context

Presently, there are multiple applied specializations situated within the broad field of psychology. Two of the historically recognized areas of specialty include industrial and organizational psychology, which focuses on the psychology of the workforce; and school psychology, which describes work with children's behavioral health and learning needs. The other two historically recognized specializations include clinical psychology and counseling psychology. The Council of Specialties in Professional Psychology (2019) formally defines clinical psychology as: "a general practice and health service provider specialty" where practitioners "assess, diagnose, predict, prevent, and treat psychopathology, mental disorders, and other individual or group problems to improve behavior adjustment, adaptation, personal effectiveness and satisfaction." Counseling psychology is formally defined as "a psychological specialty [that] facilitates personal and interpersonal functioning across the lifespan with a focus on emotional, social, work related, educational, health-related, developmental, and organizational concerns (Council of Specialties in Professional Psychology, 2019)." Each of these two applied specializations will be described in more detail in the following sections, including a brief historical overview of each.

Clinical Psychology Historical Context

Throughout much of its relatively young history, the field of psychology has focused on healing, fixing, and curing people who seek treatment for presenting mental health concerns. Following World War II, there was an increased demand for psychological services to help returning veterans, and psychologists found that agencies that funded services prioritized research into mental illness (Seligman, 2002). During this time, clinical psychology emerged as a field that employs the medical disease model, viewing mental health concerns as illnesses that demand a cure. In a descriptive article that includes the history of the medical model (or, the deficit model), Yip (2005) provided a description of some of the core assumptions of a disease orientation approach to people with psychosis (people with psychosis). Some of these key elements include: impairment of client's abilities and rights is due to their unstable mental symptoms that have the potential to harm themselves and others; relapse is due to noncompliance in medication and treatment; and the role of the therapist is the enforcer of medical compliance and social control of relapse and risk management. These features of the deficit model approach to treatment in some ways reflect the perspective of its proponents. That is, the atypical experiences of people with psychosis can be classified as an illness that requires a solution or cure. Although some mental health service consumers prefer the language of the medical model and to understand their symptoms as stemming from a disease (Steinberg & White, 1996), others do not prefer this conceptualization of their experiences (Elkins, 2009), and have less optimism for recovery when considering their symptoms part of an illness (Malla et al., 2015).

Although clinicians from a clinical psychology background may have been trained in the medical model that focuses on pathology, not all clinical psychologists adopt this approach. Positive psychology, which uses a strengths-based model (and will be detailed throughout this and the following chapter) was largely founded by professionals from a clinical background (Seligman & Csikszentmihalyi, 2000). Presently, some clinical psychologists incorporate positive psychology into their clinical work and research, proving that these two approaches are not incompatible, even if tensions exist between proponents of the medical model and advocates of strengths-based work. Operating from a deficit-oriented model for every client without considering personal preferences and individual experiences runs the risk of reinforcing a fundamental negative bias and reduces the ability to conceptualize clients from a holistic perspective.

Counseling Psychology Historical Context

As the origins of the medical model may be traced back to the end of World War II and an increased need for veteran assistance, so may the origins of the field of counseling psychology. Following the war, veterans were in need of education and employment opportunities, resulting in the rise of vocational guidance (Delgado-Romero et al., 2012). These needs, paired with the psychometric movement and study of individual differences for occupational functioning, helped form a demand for vocational guidance. These new demands, paired with the birth of the client-centered therapy movement in reaction to psychoanalytic and behavioralist schools of thought, helped give rise to counseling psychology as a field (Whiteley, 1984). This field of study and practice became officially acknowledged when the 1943 Joint Constitutional Committee of the American Psychological Association (APA) formed Division 17, a division of APA that is currently known as the Society of Counseling Psychology. Since its formation in earlier years, the field of counseling psychology continues to grow and expand its reach. Some of the core values that are identified as being integral to its profession and specialty include: (a) altruism and enhancing welfare of others, (b) facilitating positive relationships necessary for bringing about change in those seeking help, (c) integration of science and practice, (d) focus on healthy and optimal growth and development across the lifespan, (e) a holistic view of a person's social and cultural environment and emphasis on strength, resilience, and positive coping, (f) respect of human dignity and celebration of human diversity, (g) belief in social justice and social advocacy, (h) value in collaboration and multidisciplinary practice and research, and (i) a focus on strengths and coping in the context of remedial work for those seeking help (Packard, 2009). These tenets of the field of counseling psychology encourage holistic work with clients that incorporates their strengths and potential for improving their well-being. A discussion of some of this counseling psychology work that is integrated with positive psychology will be detailed towards the end of this chapter in the section on positive psychology.

Psychosis

Upon hearing the term "psychotic disorder," the first thing that many people think of is schizophrenia. However, psychotic disorders encompass a broad range of experiences that differ in terms of specific clusters of symptoms. The American Psychiatric Association Diagnostic and Statistical Manual of Mental Disorders, Fifth Edition (DSM-5) describes psychotic disorders as sharing the common features of abnormalities in at least one of the following domains: hallucinations, delusions, disorganized thinking, grossly disorganized or abnormal motor behavior, and negative symptoms (APA, 2013).

Hallucinations refer to perception-like experiences that occur in the absence of an external stimulus (APA, 2013). They are as clear and vivid as normal perceptions and are not under voluntary control. Although hallucinations may occur in any sensory modality, auditory hallucinations are the most common (APA, 2013). Auditory verbal hallucinations are usually experienced as voices that an individual perceives as being distinct from one's own thoughts. Similar to many other mental health disorder symptoms, there is not a known singular cause of how auditory verbal hallucinations are formed. Some evidence suggests there is a link between the auditory cortex and auditory verbal hallucinations, finding that people with dysfunctional auditory cortical spatial localization abilities are more susceptible to auditory verbal hallucinations (Perrin et al., 2018). Additionally, although a causal link is difficult to establish at this time, childhood trauma has been found to be a risk factor for developing auditory verbal hallucinations and other psychotic symptoms (Thomas & Longden, 2015). Because auditory verbal hallucinations are the most common form of hallucination, this symptom will be the primary focus of the present study.

Although auditory verbal hallucinations are the focus of this study, an introduction to other symptoms of psychosis is warranted. Delusions refer to fixed beliefs that are rigid and not amenable to change, even when contrary evidence is presented. They may be categorized as one of the following types of delusion: (a) persecutory (belief that one is going to be harmed or harassed), (b) referential (belief that environmental gestures or cues are directed at oneself), (c) grandiose (belief that one has exceptional abilities, wealth, or fame), (d) erotomanic (belief that another person is in love with the individual), (e) nihilistic (belief that a catastrophe will occur); and somatic (preoccupations regarding health and organ function). There are also three types of delusion that are categorized as bizarre due to the implausibility of the content. First, thought withdrawal refers to the belief that one's thoughts have been "removed" by an outside force. Second, thought insertion is the belief that thoughts are placed into an individual's mind by an outside source. Finally, delusions of control refer to the belief that one's actions are being manipulated by an outside force.

Disorganized thinking is another symptom common to the psychotic disorders. Disorganized thought may be inferred from a person's speech. It may be tangential or incoherent and impair effective communication (APA, 2013). Grossly disorganized or abnormal motor behavior is also a symptom that may be found among psychotic disorders. This may refer to behavior within one's environment that leads to difficulties in completing activities of daily living. Catatonic behavior is a type of disorganized or abnormal motor behavior with decreased reactivity to the environment (APA, 2013).

Finally, negative symptoms may be present in psychotic disorders. These are symptoms that refer to marked decreases in behavior across a number of areas, including diminished emotional expression (reductions in the expression of emotion in the face, eye contact, and speech), avolition (a decrease in self-motivated, purposeful activities), alogia (diminished speech output), anhedonia (the decreased ability to experience pleasure), and asociality (a lack of interest in social interactions). With auditory verbal hallucinations at the forefront of my research topic interest, I discovered through literature review that not all people who have these experiences are eligible for a diagnosis or even experiencing functional distress. People who fall into this category, known as "healthy voice-hearers" will be introduced next.

Healthy Voice-Hearers

Although auditory verbal hallucinations are present in a number of people eligible for a psychotic disorder diagnosis, they may also be experienced by people in the general population who do not meet diagnostic criteria for a disorder. These people are referred to in the literature as healthy voice-hearers. A meta-analysis by van Os et al. (2008) reviews the literature on psychotic symptoms that are found in non-clinical populations. This study is reviewed in greater detail in the following literature review chapter; however, a key takeaway from the meta-analysis is that the causes of psychotic disorders may be traced to the same factors that contribute to transitory or stand-alone psychotic experiences (including auditory verbal hallucinations) that are found in non-clinical populations.

Another study, by Baumeister and colleagues (2017) reviews how healthy voice-hearers may be understood on a psychosis continuum ranging from healthy controls to clinical voice-hearers. Experiencing auditory verbal hallucinations can also be viewed through either a "quasi-dimensional" (where auditory verbal hallucinations are related to distress and need for care) or "fully-dimensional" (in which auditory verbal hallucinations are not necessarily related to distress or need for care) model. A key finding was that healthy voice-hearers generally reported more positive experiences with auditory verbal hallucinations, including more positive messages, less negative self-evaluations, and greater control over the voices than their clinical voice-hearing counterparts. This study, too, is discussed in more detail in the following chapter. The existing literature on healthy voice-hearers provides some insight into the experiences of non-clinical populations who hear voices. This discussion of healthy voice-hearers can provide a normalizing factor that encourages clinicians to give great consideration before applying a diagnostic label to a client who reports these experiences and adopt a more holistic view of clients and their full range of experiences. One of the most significant barriers that many people with mental illness face, the experience of being stigmatized, is briefly reviewed next to highlight some of the difficulties clinicians should be aware of when working with people with severe mental illness, including psychosis.

Stigma

Stigma refers to the possession of an attribute that causes a person to be classified by society as being part of a "discredited" social category (Goffman, 1963). People who possess these attributes that render them discredited by society are likely to develop a mistrust of people and society at large. In his foundational discussion of stigma, Goffman (1963) identified several different categories of attributes that can cause people to experience this "othering" by the majority, including "tribal stigmas" (e.g. race, ethnicity, religion), "physical deformities" (e.g. physical disabilities), and "blemishes of character" (e.g. addiction, mental illness). People who possess one or more stigmatized identities experience differential treatment and judgment from society at large and are affected across multiple areas of functioning. Some of the negative effects that stigma can have on people with marginalized identities are reviewed in detail in the following chapter. Presently, I will provide a brief overview of one of these identities that is of interest for my study; the identity of having a psychotic disorder or experiencing symptoms typical of a psychotic disorder, including the experience of hearing voices.

Stigma Associated with Psychosis

As previously discussed, mental illness is a stigmatized identity that is widely acknowledged as such (Goffman, 1963). The deficit model, widely used in Western mental health services, labels people with mental health concerns as being "ill" and having something "wrong" with them. Many argue that the language of the medical model empowers people to blame their symptoms on a disease or illness; something that they have little or no control over (much the same as with many medical conditions). Although some people may identify with and prefer this language to describe their presenting problems, others argue that even diagnostic labeling can be a form of stigma (Yennari, 2011), or that mental illness in general may be viewed as a "blemish of character" (Goffman, 1963). This is particularly true of people who are diagnosed with disorders that are classified as severe mental illnesses (SMI). Even the labeling of "severe" places people in a category that is separate from the norm and provides a label that indicates severe malaise. People with schizophrenia and other psychotic disorders are typically classified as SMI. Along with a label that indicates their overall presentation as severe, there are additional stigmatic components that accompany a diagnosis of a psychotic disorder or psychotic symptomatology. Western society largely misunderstands and overpathologizes people with psychosis and experiences associated with psychosis. Pejorative labels such as "crazy" and "insane" are household words that are used flippantly by many. However, these words refer to stereotypical pictures of what a "crazy" person looks like, which may be someone who is speaking to themselves or seeing things that others cannot see. This normalization of using derogatory words to describe the abnormal behavior of others further perpetuates stigma that is associated with SMI, particularly psychosis.

People living with schizophrenia frequently experience multiple psychosocial difficulties. These difficulties often exacerbate or contribute to the stigma that is experienced by people with psychosis. A systematic literature review by Switaj and others (2012) provided a comprehensive review of the most common psychosocial difficulties in schizophrenia. Psychosocial difficulties were defined by the authors according to the biopsychosocial approach found in the WHO's International

Classification of Functioning, Disability and Health (World Health Organization, 2001).

They do not regard psychosocial difficulties to be direct consequences of schizophrenia;

rather, mediated by the environment in which people with schizophrenia live. The

authors, then, characterized psychosocial difficulties as impairments of mental functions

and activity limitations in domains like work, family life, and leisure activities.

Environmental factors (i.e., stigma, supportiveness of family, and personal factors like

self-confidence in overcoming difficulties) can impact psychosocial difficulties. Through

analysis of psychosocial difficulties in the literature, the authors concluded that there is a

need for a comprehensive approach to these difficulties related to schizophrenia in both

research and practice. The authors argued that psychosocial difficulties cannot be fully

understood and effectively improved in isolation. Attention should be paid to the specific

context in which psychosocial difficulties appear.

Critical Theory

Considering the negative role that stigma can play in the experiences of people

with psychosis can lead to a discussion on how these clients may be viewed as a

marginalized population. Critical theory, which will be expanded on in greater detail in

the following chapter, posits that people have the ability to transcend societally placed

constraints related to their marginalized identities (Creswell, 2013). Critical theory

literature also provides philosophers, researchers, and clinicians with the tools to help

empower marginalized people to move above and beyond the limitations placed on them

by society. When applied to psychology, a critical theory framework has the potential to

help clinicians acknowledge power differentials inherent in the therapeutic relationship, understand human behavior while accounting for contextual factors, and be more proactive in advocating for and empowering their clients (Parker, 2015). Although adopting a critical theory lens may be ideal for empowering clients, not all clinicians utilize this framework. Interventions that are presently used in the treatment of psychosis are introduced here next.

Current Treatments for Psychosis

Clinical guidelines on psychosis and schizophrenia, published by the National Institute for Health Care and Excellence (NICE) and the American Psychological Association (APA) advocate for an integrated approach to treatment that includes medication and psychotherapy (APA, 2000). Additionally, the APA guidelines state that all evidence-based approaches emphasize the value of family participation in treatment and stress the importance of working together collaboratively. Taken together, the clinical guidelines on psychosis and schizophrenia advocate for a biopsychosocial approach to treatment for people with psychosis. The biological component of this model emphasizes the benefits of incorporating antipsychotic medication into treatment planning. Antipsychotic medications significantly reduce the risk of relapse during the stable phase of schizophrenia, and often results in improvement or remission of positive psychotic symptoms (APA, 2000). Although a biopsychosocial approach is widely considered to be the ideal approach for treatment with this population, there is much debate around the psychological piece of the biopsychosocial model. Specifically, practitioners differ in their selection of psychotherapeutic interventions to treat psychosis.

Cognitive-Behavioral Therapy (CBT) for psychosis is one approach that is widely used to treat people with psychosis. CBT for psychosis interventions aim to assist individuals in identifying, monitoring, and evaluating assumptions, beliefs, and thoughts about their psychotic experiences. CBT also assists clients in examining the relationship between thoughts, emotions, and behavior (Menon et al., 2017). As an example of applying this intervention to someone with auditory hallucinations, CBT for psychosis may examine the beliefs associated with the voices (e.g., they are bad, or all-knowing) and consider alternative ways to come to terms with hearing the voices. It can also help clients change behaviors that reinforce those beliefs (for example, isolating themselves at home, or carrying out the commands by the voices). Mindfulness interventions for psychosis provide another approach to working with people with psychosis. These interventions incorporate mindfulness techniques to help clients with emotion regulation through increasing a person's comfort with fully experiencing the present moment (Khoury et al., 2013). In addition to these interventions, peer support is sometimes incorporated into treatment planning for people with psychosis. Peer support provides the opportunity for people in the community who have personal experience with a disorder to provide mentorship and support to clients seeking treatment (Chien et al., 2019).

Although there is evidence that demonstrates the effectiveness of several kinds of treatment approaches to working with people with psychosis, there are insufficient findings at present to conclude that any approach is more efficacious than the others. A more detailed discussion of the studies on CBT, mindfulness, peer support, and pharmacologic interventions for psychosis is provided in the following chapter that reviews the current literature. Although existing approaches to treating people with psychosis, including CBT, mindfulness, and peer support interventions include components of increasing clients' skills for symptom management, they lack an incorporation of utilizing a client's strengths, and focus primarily on symptom reduction.

Meaning-Making

One emerging area of interest in the literature on psychosis involves therapists helping clients to make sense and meaning of their experiences, including hearing voices. The goal of engaging in meaning-making processes is to help the client not merely cope with the voices, but to help them increase their sense of agency and self-worth, while providing hope for the future (Roe & Davidson, 2005). Meaning-making processes can involve encouraging proactive coping (Roe et al., 2006), helping the client enhance social functioning, and helping them engage in productive, meaningful work (Dilks et al., 2012). Although the existing literature on meaning-making processes is somewhat limited, specific studies are outlined in detail in the following chapter. Presently, I will shift to a discussion on the positive psychology movement, which incorporates elements of meaning-making into clinical work.

Positive Psychology

Positive psychology is a movement that emerged in response to the deficit-based perspectives that have been adopted by the medical model and widely used in psychology. In their introductory article on positive psychology, Seligman and Csikszentmihaly (2000) argue that psychology is not merely the study of pathology, weakness, and damage; rather, it also is the study of strength and virtue found within people. Treatment shifts from a focus on fixing what is broken to nurturing strengths to help people reach their potential and thrive. Clients have a more collaborative role in their treatment. Rather than acting as passive recipients of mental health services, they are viewed as active decision-makers who may make meaning of their experiences and have choices, preferences, and possibilities in the course of their treatment. The positive psychology movement challenges the medical model's underlying belief that the absence of symptoms is sufficient for optimal mental health (Drvaric et al., 2015). Instead, there is a shift from clinical recovery to personal recovery, which uses an individual's strengths to help cultivate meaning in life, as well as building adaptive attitudes, values, feelings, goals, and skills. A core belief underlying this movement is that people have the potential to flourish, even amid the presence of symptoms of mental illness, including psychosis (Slade, 2010).

Counseling psychology shares considerable overlap with some of the core principles of positive psychology, primarily, a focus on client strengths, assets, and potentialities regardless of the degree of psychopathology (APA, 1999; Gelso & Fretz, 2001; Savickas, 2003). The APA Society of Counseling Psychology has a section within the division that is devoted to positive psychology. As part of the section's purpose statement, the Section on Positive Psychology identifies an aim to encourage contributions to research and practice in positive psychology by Division 17 members. The section identifies goals that include: (a) continuing to define and promote positive psychology within and outside of counseling psychology; (b) bringing together counseling psychologists who have an interest in positive psychology; (c) promoting the integration of science and practice in positive psychology; (d) promoting positive psychology within the field of psychology and the public sphere; (e) helping to define, promote, and support the education of counseling psychologists interested in positive psychology; (f) supporting, encouraging, and promoting links between Section members and other related specialties; (g) developing and sponsoring programs related to positive psychology to be presented at conventions; (h) recognizing outstanding contributions of members; (i) posting a membership directory to facilitate networking among members; and (j) developing resources to assist with training and research in positive psychology. The formation and maintenance of this society demonstrates an ongoing interest in practitioners with counseling psychology backgrounds using a strengths-based perspective and other elements of positive psychology in their practice. Also, overlap between positive psychology and counseling psychology was examined in a content analysis by Lopez et al. (2006). This study is further detailed in the following chapter, but a key takeaway is that throughout history, counseling psychology has incorporated positive elements into its work, and can benefit as a field through continuing to strengthen this connection.

Positive Psychology Interventions

A key practical implication present in the positive psychology literature is that clinicians should emphasize a client's goals and strengths and integrate this information with interventions that promote well-being. Positive psychology interventions are therapeutic treatments that facilitate the effective use of a person's strengths to solve problems and build resilience (Drvaric et al., 2015). Some researchers have suggested that clients with schizophrenia can benefit from enhancing their well-being and building strengths (Meyer et al., 2012), because increased well-being and building strengths are associated with longer periods between relapse and symptom improvement (Fava & Tomba, 2009). Positive psychotherapy interventions focus on working with people with psychosis towards personal recovery that goes beyond the removal of psychotic symptoms. Rather, recovery is different for every client, and is meaningfully defined by each individual according to their personal needs and goals (Meyer et al., 2012). Themes that emerge in terms of personal recovery include hope and optimism, self-determination and self-respect, coping and openness to discovery and new experiences (Ralph, 2000). Recovery should extend beyond the removal of symptoms, which often lead to remission but do not always result in improvements that ultimately result in recovery. Positive psychotherapy interventions target a client's well-being while at the same time building strengths and resources that can help an individual with symptom management.

Practitioner Perspectives of Psychosis

There has been growing interest in recent years in learning about how people with psychosis understand and make meaning of their psychotic experiences; however, little attention has been paid to investigating mental health practitioners' beliefs about people with psychosis. One study that was conducted by Carter et al. (2017) began to investigate this topic through a review of practitioners' beliefs about the etiology of psychosis, the treatment offered to clients with psychosis, and the effectiveness of these treatments. Carter et al. (2017) found that clinicians support a combination of psychosocial and pharmacologic treatment in working with people with psychosis, which is consistent with the biopsychosocial approach advocated by the NICE (2014) guidelines for psychosis interventions. However, the specific methods that clinicians favored using with this population differed according to therapists' training experiences and therapeutic orientations. Many participants in this study reported having limited training in working with psychosis. The study by Carter and others (2017) as well as the NICE (2014) guidelines for psychosis are described in more detail in a literature review presented in the following chapter. However, these studies are part of a small sample of research in this area. A key takeaway is that there is currently a lack of literature that describes mental health practitioners' views of and experiences with working with people with psychosis.

Statement of the Problem

There is a lack of research on clinicians' beliefs and understanding of people with who hear voices, specifically regarding their = of clients who have psychotic experiences, treatment planning with these clients, and the prognoses for these clients.

Significance of the Problem

Research that explores mental health practitioners' beliefs about and experiences who hear voices is needed for multiple reasons. Although there has been a growing interest in learning about the experiences of people who hear voices directly from this population, there is a lack of understanding about how clinicians understand and work with their clients who have these experiences. In addition, the positive psychology movement is still relatively young. The existing literature could benefit from phenomenological research from a critical theory framework that explores practitioners' views of and experiences with people who hear voices through a positive psychology lens.

Purpose of the Study

There is a need for research on therapists' experiences of working with people who hear voices and their view of clients in the context of a strengths-based perspective. The purpose of this investigation is to address how psychologists and psychology trainees presently conceptualize their clients who hear voices and investigate for any variables that comprise a strengths-based perspective. Providing a greater understanding of practitioners' views of people who hear voices and how they treat these clients can provide crucial information about the current landscape of mental health services and how clients with these experiences are viewed in terms of treatment planning and prognoses. For this project, when referring to questions about participants' clients, the terms "people with psychosis" or "clients with psychosis" will be used to describe clients who experience a psychotic disorder, while "people who hear voices" will be used as a more broad term that does not necessitate a diagnosis.

Research Questions

Specifically, this qualitative phenomenological study will use a critical theory framework and will explore clinicians' interview responses for themes that relate to a positive psychology or strengths-based approach. The broad, central research question will be: How do psychologists and psychology trainees conceptualize and plan work with clients who hear voices? Specific research sub-questions stem from this central theme, and may be broken down as follows: (a) What are the experiences of clinicians in working with people with psychosis, specifically, people who experience hearing voices? (b) How do clinicians approach treatment planning with clients who hear voices? (c) How do clinicians feel about working with people who hear voices? Specifically, how do they think their own views affect their work with these clients; how do they feel that their clients may be affected by biases of others? Are they familiar with critical theory? (d) Are clinicians familiar with healthy voice-hearers? What do they believe differentiates healthy voice-hearers from people with psychosis? (e) How do psychologists and psychology trainees believe that their doctoral program (both education and training) prepared them for working with people who hear voices? (f) To what degree do clinicians incorporate elements of positive psychology in their beliefs, experiences, and treatment planning of clients who experience hearing voices? (g) What do practitioners believe recovery looks like for people who hear voices?

Description of the Study

To address the research questions, this qualitative study employed an empirical phenomenological methodology guided by a critical theory framework that acknowledges people with psychosis and people who hear voices as a marginalized population. Although the sample consisted of clinicians, the ultimate subjects of this study were clients with which participants described their work. Many of these clients were in the maintenance, rather than acute, phase of psychosis, and experienced symptoms that aligned with the mild, rather than severe, end of the psychosis continuum. The sample for this study was recruited from multiple local mental health settings and consisted of psychologists and psychology trainees with training backgrounds in clinical and counseling psychology. Participants were interviewed using a protocol (attached in Appendix A) that followed a semi-structured interview format and asked questions to learn about the essence of their experiences in working with people who hear voices. The procedures for data collection and analysis are detailed in Chapter 3.

Significance of the Study

This study has the potential to benefit both practitioners and clients of mental health services in several ways. It can add to the sparse existing literature on clinicians' views of working with people with psychosis. This research can provide practitioners with an opportunity to learn about how others in their field of practice view people with psychosis as well as healthy voice-hearers, which can enhance their awareness of biases that may be present in working with people who report what may be characterized as a psychotic symptom. Learning about the biases of others can encourage practitioners to view their own biases that may be present when working with both people with psychosis and healthy voice-hearers. This study will also highlight elements of the positive psychology framework that practitioners may use when conceptualizing and working with clients, leaving implications for how practitioners may consider integrating a strengths-based approach into their work.

This study can also provide training implications for doctoral programs across multiple disciplines. Speaking to participants can provide more information about the strengths (e.g., positive psychology education, education on psychosis and experiences of hearing voices) that practitioners from both counseling and clinical psychology identified in their training programs. Including participants from both disciplines can allow for rich perspectives that psychologists and psychology trainees have to offer, and can allow them the opportunity to speak about how their education and training impacted their work with clients who hear voices.

Finally, in addition to impacting clinicians and training programs, this study has the potential to improve the treatment that people with psychosis and healthy voice-hearers experience. Highlighting the use of a strengths-based approach in understanding and working with these clients can lead to more individual empowerment through experiences of more acceptance and less stigmatization in the mental health community. This study has the potential to positively impact people who experience psychotic symptoms, including those who meet criteria for a psychotic disorder diagnosis as well as those who report hearing voices as an experience exclusive of other psychosis symptoms.

This may be accomplished through practical implications which include increased

awareness at the client, service provider, and training program levels.

CHAPTER II

LITERATURE REVIEW

In Chapter 2, I provide an extensive review of the extant literature that will help inform my approach to my research topic. My proposed research involves learning from both clinical-and counseling-trained psychologists and psychology trainees about their experiences working with people who hear voices, with attention to elements of a strengths-based perspective that clinicians may use with this population. In a style similar to Chapter 1, I outline this section by topics, opening with a review of the literature on stigma in general, then of stigma associated with severe mental health diagnoses, including psychotic disorders. Following the discussion on stigma, I provide an introduction to critical theory and how people with severe mental illness symptoms (including auditory verbal hallucinations) may be viewed as having a marginalized identity. Next, I share information about healthy voice-hearers and the characteristics that distinguish "healthy" people who hear voices from people who share these experiences but meet diagnostic criteria for a psychotic disorder. Current treatments for people with psychosis are then reviewed, with a focus on CBT and mindfulness interventions for psychosis, as well as approaches that involve clinicians helping clients make meaning of their experiences, particularly regarding hearing voices. This topic then leads to a discussion of positive psychology, including positive psychology interventions and the applications they may have when working with people who hear voices. Finally, practitioners' perspectives on people with psychosis are reviewed. Throughout each of these sections, current empirical studies are detailed and discussed within the broader context of each topic. Gaps in the literature are identified as well, particularly in regard to learning about therapists' views of people with psychosis, particularly through a positive psychology-informed perspective. Other areas for research that will be discussed include learning about training for counseling psychologists, and the lack of discussion on psychosis-related symptoms (primarily, auditory verbal hallucinations, both for clinical and non-clinical people) in education.

Stigma

The effects of stigma can increase difficulties across multiple areas of life for people who have at least one marginalized identity. Lamb et al. (2011) conducted a qualitative meta-synthesis of studies with some of these groups of people to understand how stigma creates barriers to accessing health care. In their analysis, twenty qualitative studies were identified across six databases, consisting of 531 participants who were categorized in one of the following areas: (a) people suffering from advanced cancer, (b) adolescents with eating disorders, (c) asylum seekers and refugees, (d) people from black and ethnic minority groups, (e) depressed elderly people, (f) long-term unemployed people, (g) homeless people, and (h) people with medically unexplained symptoms.

In their analysis of the studies, Lamb et al. (2011) extracted first- and second-order concepts, both preserving interpretations of experiences from the original participants and preserving interpretations from the original studies' authors, then they developed third-order concepts through their own interpretations of the synthesized data. They found that stigma emerged as a theme across the studies, specifically, people experienced judgment and discrimination from others daily due to their physical appearance or social position. They regularly perceived, expected, and often experienced this discrimination due to their identity when seeking health care, and believed their mental health problems to be rooted in social problems. These findings highlight the significant impact that social stigma can have on people with a stigmatized identity, including presenting limitations to seeking health care.

Stigma can be especially impactful for people who have multiple, intersecting marginalized identities. The experiences of stigma related to some of these intersecting identities was explored through a systematic review of the literature on stigma experienced by people with HIV/AIDS, mental illness, and physical disability. Jackson-Best and Edwards (2018) searched five electronic databases to search for reviews published between 2005 and 2017 that addressed their research topic on intersectionality among people with these identities. In total, 98 reviews (including integrative reviews, quantitative systematic reviews, meta-analyses, and qualitative systematic reviews) were selected for Jackson-Best and Edwards' (2018) review. The authors provided a cross-analysis of the selected reviews, and discovered that, although stigma attached to more than one identity was discussed in each reviewed article, few articles ($n = 13$) used an intersectional lens to analyze primary research studies, and even fewer ($n = 3$) provided a definition of intersectionality. Although they were few in number, these reviews described how mental illness or and HIV/AIDS diagnosis intersected with culture, power, and other contextual factors to reinforce social conditions that perpetuate stigma.

Another demonstration of people with marginalized identities facing stigma can be seen through a systematic review and qualitative meta-synthesis by Vanstone et al. (2017). Here, challenges to diet modification were examined in both marginalized and non-marginalized adults with diabetes. A systematic review of primary qualitative studies (= 120) was conducted, using studies, published from 2002-2015 across three databases. Through a qualitative meta-synthesis, these original studies were synthesized through a staged coding process, where findings were thematically categorized. Multiple marginalized identities were found across the studies, including minority ethnicity ($n =$ 58), low SES ($n = 31$), female gender ($n = 15$), rural population status ($n = 12$), old age ($n = 21$), and physical disability ($n = 2$).

Vanstone et al. (2017) found that social marginalization and the stigma of being marginalized contributed to increased difficulty in diet modification through problems with self-discipline, emotions, family and social support, knowledge and significance of food, and knowledge and information. Essentially, the stigma associated with social marginalization intersects with the stigma of diabetes and exacerbates the barriers to diet modification. This study as well as the meta-analysis by Jackson-Best and Edwards (2018) provide a glimpse into the compounding negative effects that stigma of marginalized identities has on people's well-being across numerous areas of life. People with severe mental disorders (SMI), including psychosis often experience stigma and may be viewed as a marginalized population using a critical theory lens. Stigma and marginalization experienced by people with psychosis will be highlighted next.

Stigma Associated with Psychosis

People with severe mental disorders make up a large part of the population that receives treatment through mental health services, but they receive less focus and understanding from both providers and the general population than those diagnosed with the more common mood disorders, such as anxiety and depressive disorders (Li et al., 2019). In addition, the very label that is applied to people with more severe presenting concerns (SMI) distinguishes people with these disorders as being separate, more severe and in need of more intensive care than people who seek treatment for a less severe disorder. This language may be viewed as a way in which diagnostic labeling continues to perpetuate stigma in people with mental health concerns that include psychosis. Psychotic experiences that are present in the psychotic disorders commonly involve delusions as well as auditory and visual hallucinations. People who experience these symptoms and meet criteria for a psychotic disorder are given the diagnostic label of "psychotic" or "schizophrenic" that carries with it a stigma; complete with shame, behavioral expectations, and fear of the unknown (Li et al., 2019). This labeling has the effect of "othering" people with psychosis, because they are marked and identified as deviating from the non-psychotic normative population (Randal et al., 2009). The World Health Organization (WHO) has made efforts as part of an anti-stigma campaign to provide psychoeducation around SMI. In these efforts, separate but interacting vicious cycles have been identified for the individual, the family, and the mental health services that create and perpetuate stigma. These cycles exacerbate disability and feelings of helplessness for people with psychosis, as well as increase difficulties for their families and mental health care providers. Stigma can create a significant barrier to obtaining mental health services (Gronholm et al., 2017). For people with psychosis, this obstacle can be particularly problematic; as timely access to treatment is associated with improved outcomes in this population (Birchwood & Macmillan, 1993; McGorry & Yung, 1996). Several studies will be reviewed here that illustrate ways that stigma in people with psychosis has been examined in current research.

A systematic review by Gronholm et al. (2017) evaluated findings from studies that include qualitative, quantitative, and mixed-method research that examined the relationship between stigma and pathways to care with people with first-episode psychosis or those at a clinically-defined risk for developing a psychotic disorder. The researchers used five electronic databases to search for papers published between 1996 and 2016. Forty articles were ultimately selected for inclusion in this meta-synthesis, including 31 qualitative, seven quantitative, and two mixed-methods studies. The researchers synthesized data in three stages: thematic analysis, narrative synthesis, and a meta-synthesis. The thematic analysis involved synthesizing the findings of articles reporting qualitative data using NVivo, a type of qualitative analysis software. Inductive open coding was used to index and sort themes, resulting in a thematic framework that reflected the data. The second stage of narrative synthesis involved the authors assessing quantitative findings across the studies about stigma and pathways to care and summarizing them within a textual narrative. Finally, the third stage of analysis involved a meta-synthesis in which the researchers combined the findings of both the qualitative and quantitative syntheses. The themes that were identified through these processes included: (a) sense of difference, (b) characterizing differences negatively, (c) negative reactions (anticipated and experienced), (d) strategies; (e) lack of knowledge and understanding, and (f) service-related factors.

Through the quantitative studies that were analyzed with narrative synthesis, the authors found an increase in perceived stigma among people at risk for psychosis between baseline and one-year follow-up being associated with more negative help-seeking attitudes at follow-up. The less stigma stress an individual had, the more they were likely to have positive help-seeking attitudes towards both psychotherapy and medication use. Overall, they found close coherence between the qualitative and quantitative evidence; finding that quantitative results fit within the themes that emerged from the qualitative synthesis. The quality of all examined studies' methodology was assessed using the Mixed Methods Appraisal Tool (Pluye et al., 2011) and was found to be acceptable. The Mixed Methods Appraisal Tool assessed core quality criteria and methodology-specific aspects that include four quality dimensions for quantitative and qualitative study designs, and three dimensions for mixed-methods designs. Researchers using this tool assigned one point for each dimension that was met for each article, and half of a point for each dimension where criteria were partially met The points were then totaled for an overall score. Gronholm and others (2017) only used articles that met at least 50% of Mixed Methods Appraisal Tool criteria for their meta-synthesis. The forty studies included in the synthesis were determined to be methodologically sound, as they met at least 50% of the appraisal tool's criteria. A major conclusion of this study is that stigma can serve as a barrier to engaging in help-seeking behavior, particularly for first-episode psychosis or at-risk for psychotic disorder individuals. Clinical implications include mental health awareness efforts focusing on increasing the understanding of early signs of psychosis, and improving awareness of how to interpret early symptoms to reduce barriers to help-seeking behaviors.

Next, I will review several studies that were included in the meta-synthesis by Gronholm and colleagues (2017). Each of these studies focuses on stigma experienced by people with psychosis and highlights the problematic nature of stigma for people in this population.

The first of these studies is a quantitative study by Rusch and others (2013). I selected this study for review due to the evidence it presents for a relationship between stigmas that people with psychosis face and their negative attitudes towards therapy. This cross-sectional study collected data from 176 Swiss participants who met criteria for being high-risk for psychosis based on scores on the Schizophrenia Proneness Interview (Schultze-Lutte et al., 2007), or the Structured Interview for Prodromal Syndromes (Miller et al., 2003). Similar to the measures used by Xu and others (2016), these researchers measured: (a) stigma stress using the Stigma Stress Scale (Rusch et al., 2009), (b) perceived stress using the Perceived Devaluation-Discrimination Questionnaire (Link, 1987), and (c) positive and negative symptoms using the PANSS (Kay et al., 1987). The researchers found positive attitudes towards psychotherapy to be significantly associated with lower stigma stress ($B = -0.29$, $t = -3.19$, $p > .05$) and negative symptoms ($B = -0.27$, $t = -3.07$, $p > .05$). Although this cross-sectional analysis does not provide evidence of causality, it does highlight a relationship between stigma and negative attitudes that people with psychosis have towards therapy.

Xu et al. (2016) explored perceived stigma and stigma stress as predictors of attitudes towards psychotherapy among young people at risk for psychosis. This study was a follow-up to the above-described article published by Rusch and colleagues (2013). Data from the sixty-seven participants used in the Rusch et al. (2013) study was collected at follow-up by Xu and others (2016). These participants completed the Perceived Devaluation-Discrimination Questionnaire (Link, 1987) to measure their perceived public stigma; the Stigma Stress Scale (Rusch et al., 2009) to measure their personal appraisal of stigma they experience; and the PANSS (Kay et al., 1987) to measure positive and negative symptoms. These measures were completed both at baseline during Rusch and others' study (2013) and at one-year follow-up. Using multiple linear regressions, Xu and colleagues (2016) found that baseline levels of perceived stigma, stigma stress, and clinical symptoms did not predict attitudes towards medication and psychotherapy at one-year follow-up. However, they did find that an increase of perceived stigma ($B = -.28$, $t = -2.26$, $p < .05$), stigma stress ($B = -0.30$, $t = -2.35$, $p < .05$), and positive symptoms ($B = -0.35$, $t = -2.54$, $p < .05$) predicted more negative attitudes towards psychotherapy at follow-up. A key takeaway from this study is that perceived stigma and stigma stress may contribute to resistance to seeking psychotherapy for people with psychosis and those at risk for psychosis.

Qualitative studies can also provide insight into how stigma is experienced by people with psychosis, and several were included in the meta-synthesis by Gronholm et al. (2017). One of these studies that provides insight into the experience of stigma by people with psychosis is an exploratory and inductive qualitative study that explored delays in help-seeking behavior for people who had experienced first-episode psychosis. Ferrari and others (2015) used 34 participants (25 people who experienced first-episode psychosis, and nine family members) to explore similarities and differences in pathways to care and the duration of psychosis that was left untreated across African-origin, Caribbean-origin, and European-origin groups. Data were collected through focus groups and analyzed using thematic analysis to identify themes. To establish rigor and trustworthiness in their study, Ferrari et al. (2015) used multiple data sources in their analysis (e.g., pathways maps from semi-structured interviews, chart reviews, focus group data) and engaged in team debriefing.

One key finding from this study was a discussion of stigma affecting help-seeking behaviors across narratives in all focus groups. Participants experienced more internalized stigma about psychosis if their family members held negative views of people with psychosis. Differences between physical and mental illness also emerged relating to this theme; people acknowledged family members would be more supportive of a physical illness than they would a mental illness, especially psychosis. One difference that was found among groups were factors contributing to stigma. Participants in the African-origin and Caribbean-origin groups explained religious beliefs as contributing to their internalized stigma (e.g., believing psychosis was a punishment from God); this finding was not present in the European-origin group. Regarding help-seeking behavior, participants across groups reported withholding information about their auditory verbal hallucinations when working with a healthcare provider who they perceived as having negative attitudes towards psychosis. Ten participants reported that general practitioners were their first point of contact in their pathways to care; nine of these participants received misdiagnoses or had their symptoms dismissed by these providers.

Although this study used a small sample of participants that was limited to three ethnicities, it does highlight differences that are prevalent across cultures in terms of barriers to seeking help for psychosis. Additionally, an important takeaway from this study is that stigma from the environment (e.g., family support, religious influence, health care providers' opinions) can substantially contribute to a person's internalized stigma and in turn affect their likelihood of seeking treatment.

Another qualitative study that provides information on help-seeking behaviors related to psychosis is a case study approach by Boydell et al. (2013). Similar to the study by Ferrari and colleagues (2015), this research focused on help-seeking pathways. The sample used for this study consisted of ten young people in Canada (ranging from ages 14-20) who met criteria for ultra-high-risk for psychosis, per Criteria of Prodromal Symptoms criteria. Data collected included two interviews with each participant (spaced 2-10 months apart), interviews with significant others of these participants, and field notes from the interviews. Thematic analyses of the data revealed that young people were often active in initiating help-seeking behaviors, rather than being influenced by parents, teachers, or others to begin treatment. Stigma was found to be a significant factor in the delay of seeking help. Several participants' case studies reflected an unwillingness to discuss mental illness with family members, even if there was a history of mental illness in the family. As with the findings from Ferrari et al., this collection of case studies demonstrates the detrimental role that stigma frequently plays in impeding help-seeking behavior for people with psychosis.

In an empirical phenomenological study, Yennari (2011) interviewed seven people with a schizophrenia diagnosis about their lived experiences and perceptions (of self and of self by others) of living with the disorder. Using the empirical phenomenological method, Yennari (2011) provided detailed information about each step of data collection and analysis so that the study may be replicated. She used reflexive procedures of acknowledging a priori assumptions, researcher reflections, and explicating implicit assumptions, and finally analyzed the findings in light of a priori assumptions. Using the empirical phenomenology approach, these researcher presuppositions were not viewed as an obstacle, but as key to the results, and useful in forming a frame of reference from which the phenomenon could be understood (Walsh, 2004).

Themes that emerged were grouped under two clusters: (a) issue of living with the diagnostic label (label on identity, concealment of label, facing ignorance and stigma), and (b) experiences specific to schizophrenia (onset, role in spirituality with coping, tension of trust/mistrust, medication compliance/noncompliance, and perceptions of unhelpful and beneficial aspects of treatment). Regarding the unhelpful aspects of treatment that participants in this study reported, many people felt they had a loss of freedom and control over their treatment, particularly in the hospital setting. This feeling was often exacerbated by treatment providers who participants perceived as being uncaring and not taking patients seriously. Conversely, participants reported positive experiences with mental health providers when they reported working with staff who they described as "caring, empathetic" as well as authentically listening to the patients. Although the small sample size ($n = 7$) of this study may limit the generalizability of the findings, the phenomenological method the researcher employed provided insight into some shared factors in the experiences of people with schizophrenia, while inviting future researchers to expand on phenomenological data collection with this population.

As the literature presented here illustrates, people with psychosis can have experiences with stigma that can lead to understanding them as a marginalized group. In addition to stigma, people with psychosis often experience barriers to treatment that reflect clinicians' biases towards these clients' clinical presentations. Although literature on clinicians viewing people with psychosis as a marginalized group appears to be sparse, other literature shows that therapists may be resistant to working with this population. The NICE (2010) guidelines on schizophrenia and psychosis provide guidance to therapists to refer clients with psychosis to a higher level of care (e.g., crisis resolution, home treatment team) if they present with symptoms of early psychosis. Although these guidelines were developed to align with clients' best interests, there is a risk of clinicians making referrals without full consideration of multiple factors that make up clients' experiences. For example, some people experience auditory verbal hallucinations without any distress or other symptoms of psychosis. These individuals may be referred to as healthy voice-hearers and are introduced with more detail in a following section. First, however, the discussion on how clinicians may conceptualize people with psychosis as a marginalized population will be continued through a critical theory lens.

Critical Theory

Critical theory is a framework that empowers people to transcend constraints that are socially placed upon those with stigmatized identities (Creswell, 2013). Critical race theory was an important predecessor to the broader movement of critical theory. Critical race theory examines intersectionality of race, legal, and social issues, and emphasizes how structural forces perpetuate racial inequities (Crenshaw et al., 1995). There is current discourse about critical race theory at the time of writing this paper, in light of the political and social climate present in the United States, including racial injustices that have been increasingly in the news. A current example of people applying critical theory to a movement is the Academics for Black Survival and Wellness, a group of academics who aim to honor the toll of racial trauma for Black people and educate Non-Black academics about these realities and how they can initiate change (Academics for Black Survival and Wellness, 2021). This group offers anti-racism training, which provides academics with an understanding of historical and systemic inequities, intersectionality, Whiteness in academia, and how to practice Black allyship and advocate for changes in academia and beyond.

Another current application of critical theory to a movement can be found through critical disability theory (Hosking, 2008). Proponents of critical disability theory consider this framework to be a theoretical approach to the concept of disability that rejects a deficits-based view and instead proposes several social-based principles. These include: (a) disability is a social construct instead of an impairment consequence; (b) disability can be viewed as a complex intersectionality of impairment, individual responses, and the social environment; and (c) social disadvantages of disability are caused by the social environment. Critical disability theorists emphasize that the environmental conditions of present-day society are not designed to meet the needs of people with disabilities, and changes must be made at structural levels to accommodate all people as well as redefine the concept of normalcy and ability (Hosking, 2008).

Understanding people with psychosis as being part of a marginalized population can increase clinicians' awareness of additional difficulties that their clients may face in daily life. A critical theory framework may be adopted by therapists to more deeply understand this marginalized identity that their clients may have, while enabling them to empower these clients and move towards a greater societal understanding of psychosis. Researchers and practitioners who are guided by a critical theory lens in their research and understanding of clients acknowledge that power and oppression are key issues in the experiences of marginalized groups (Merriam, 2009). Given the stigma that many people with psychosis experience, clinicians who adopt a critical theory perspective may be more equipped to engage in advocacy as well as help their clients advocate for themselves. Several of the studies reviewed in the section on stigma included data from participants who were in acute inpatient settings or experiencing first-episode or otherwise acute psychosis (e.g., Boydell et al., 2013; Ferrari et al., 2015; Gronholm et al., 2017). People who experience first-episode or acute psychosis, as well as those who experience more severe psychosis symptoms, may be considered at higher risk for stigma due to societal misunderstandings about psychosis. As they prepare their advocacy and empowerment efforts, clinicians can be aware that people on different levels of the continuum of psychosis (Baumeister et al., 2017) may experience different levels of stigma with unique challenges, including biases from healthcare providers who may lack exposure to clients with these experiences.

Critical psychology is a psychological perspective that has foundations in critical theory (Parker, 2015). As with critical theory, critical psychology transcends mainstream explanations of problems, emphasizes contextual factors and oppressive environmental constraints, and advocates for progressive social change that empowers marginalized groups. Proponents of critical psychology challenge the conventional knowledge of the field, calling attention to mainstream psychology for not acknowledging the influences of power differentials between groups (Parker, 2015). More specifically, a criticism of the field is that researchers and clinicians tend to explain human behavior at an individual level without accounting for multiple contextual factors.

One main concept that exists in critical psychology is the psy-complex, the notion that psychological sciences maintain the social order and status quo, and fail to recognize that power differentials in daily life continue to be upheld (e.g., schools, prisons, hospitals) (Castel et al., 1982). Proponents of the psy-complex argue that the different disciplines found within the social sciences maintain the aforementioned power differential by remaining divided and functioning as separate entities (Rose, 1985). Critical psychologists advocate for linking the social science disciplines and activities and encouraging professionals to engage in theoretical debate and challenge the generally accepted norms of their disciplines. Multiple practical implications stem from critical psychology's notion of the psy-complex, but these implications appear to be mostly for researchers and less for practitioners. For example, Martinussen (2018, p. 9) suggests that researchers "keep disciplinary bounds porous"and actively seek out researchers from social science disciplines other than their own.

Although critical theory (and, more specifically, critical psychology and the notion of the psy-complex) continues to be used by researchers as a guiding framework for scholarly discussions and theoretical publications, there appears to be sparse empirical literature that uses critical theory to explore the experiences of people with severe mental health experiences, specifically, psychotic symptoms. Critical theory as a guiding framework for the present study will be further explored in the following chapter. As I continue my literature review, I will next discuss the experiences of one symptom generally associated with psychosis (auditory verbal hallucinations) and its prevalence in otherwise healthy individuals.

Healthy Voice-Hearers

The tendency to pathologize experiences such as auditory verbal hallucinations as psychotic symptoms is common among mental health practitioners (Longden & Waterman, 2012). Although these experiences can be one symptom present among others in a typical diagnostic profile of a psychotic disorder (such as schizophrenia), the experience of hearing voices is not necessarily exclusive to people who meet diagnostic criteria for a psychotic disorder. Several studies outlined below discuss the experiences of people who are considered healthy; not meeting diagnostic criteria for a psychotic or other mental disorder, but who experience hearing voices. These people are referred to in the literature as healthy voice-hearers.

A meta-analysis by van Os and colleagues (2008) covered all reported incidence and prevalence studies of population rates of subclinical psychotic experiences at the time of the study. The authors began by defining a psychosis continuum; it implies that clinical psychotic symptoms can be found in non-clinical populations as well. The overarching assumption of the continuum approach to psychosis is that experiencing symptoms of psychosis is not necessarily associated with the presence of the disorder. They also made a distinction between subclinical population psychotic experiences vs. subclinical psychotic symptoms; the symptoms are associated with distress and help-seeking behavior, but do not always result in psychotic disorder. Thus, there is a cut-off between psychotic symptoms and a psychotic disorder. The authors reviewed articles from the Medline database, spanning from 1950-2007. For the meta-analysis, 47 articles were selected that met inclusion criteria, which were that selected studies must have: (a) reported on a study of a general population sample with complete data on a minimum of 100 participants, (b) included incidence or prevalence rates for dichotomous psychosis outcomes, and (c) been published as original research in or after 1950. To summarize the rate data, the researchers used the graphical approach to the analysis of epidemiological findings (Saha et al., 2008), which displays variations in frequency estimates rather than collapsing data into one pooled estimate.

Among the findings, van Os and colleagues (2008) suggested subclinical psychotic experiences are mostly transitory; prevalent but with good outcomes, although a small proportion do continue to develop a psychotic disorder. Additional environmental risk factors can (e.g., trauma, urbanicity, and cannabis use) can result in poorer outcomes. Transitory developmental expression of psychosis has the potential to persist abnormally, thus becoming clinically relevant depending on the degree of environmental risk that the individual is exposed to additionally. This may be understood as part of the proneness – persistence – impairment model of the onset of psychotic disorder. In summary, the causes of a psychotic disorder may be traced to the same factors that make the common, transitory developmental expression of subclinical psychosis persist. This highlights the importance of clinical efforts to detect and intervene at an earlier stage; as well as the fact that psychotic experiences, including auditory verbal hallucinations, do not exclusively occur within clinical populations, and may be experienced by people who are considered healthy.

A comprehensive literature review by Baumeister, Sedgwick, Howes, and Peters (2017) examined research on healthy individuals who experienced auditory verbal hallucinations but did not express distress or a need for care. The purpose of this review was to examine how healthy voice-hearers were conceptualized regarding the diagnostic vs. "quasi-" and "fully-dimensional" continuum models of psychosis. Thirty-six articles selected from three databases (PsycINFO, EMBASE, and Medline) were used in this review. The authors opened the review by claiming there to be accumulating evidence that the experience of auditory verbal hallucination (auditory verbal hallucinations) is not necessarily uncommon in healthy individuals, and therefore is not always an indicator of psychopathology. They reminded the reader that auditory verbal hallucinations are present in a range of mental disorders (e.g., depression, anxiety, posttraumatic stress disorder [PTSD], obsessive compulsive disorder [OCD]). They then introduced the continuum model; the argument against diagnostic classification by category, and towards a shift of experiences that extends beyond clinical populations to the general public. According to the continuum model, healthy voice-hearers are situated between clinical voice-hearers and healthy controls. The two major conceptualizations of the continuum model are quasi-dimensional (in which psychotic experiences are thought to be directly related to distress and need for care) and fully dimensional (in which occurrences of psychotic experiences is not necessarily related to distress or need for care).

The review found that across all studies, negative content of the voices' messages was found in clinical voice-hearers but not healthy voice-hearers. Healthy voice-hearers experienced positive messages, such as advice-giving. Healthy voice-hearers heard fewer negative evaluations about themselves from the voices, but more comments making evaluations of others (Honig et al., 1998; Kravik et al., 2015). All studies reviewed by the researchers found that healthy voice-hearers reported little to no voice-related distress, or that distress was significantly lower than clinical voice-hearers. Many studies found healthy voice-hearers reported greater control over voices, and one study found that healthy status was predicted by: (a) high control over voices, (b) low frequency of voices, (c) age of onset before 16, and (d) mostly positive voice content (Daalman et al., 2011). Negative experiences were predicted by: (a) negative voice content, (b) more voices arguing with each other or talking all at once, (c) voices remarking on the individual, and (d) disturbing contact with other people (Beavan & Read, 2010). More than 90% of healthy voice-hearers reported no disturbance to their life by auditory verbal hallucinations (Sommer et al., 2010). Spirituality and auditory verbal hallucinations were also examined in both groups; healthy voice-hearers who identified as religious experienced significantly more positive perceptions of voices than non-religious healthy voice-hearers and clinical voice-hearers (Davies et al., 2001). Taylor and Murray (2012) found that initial voice distress was mitigated by the person engaging with the voices and integrating them into a spiritual framework. All studies that considered trauma as a variable found that increased trauma exposure is similar for healthy and clinical voice-hearers. In what the authors called an interesting finding, healthy voice-hearers were significantly less likely to identify their stressful life events as related to auditory verbal hallucination onset, compared with clinical voice-hearers.

Next, several key studies included in Baumeister et al.'s (2017) comprehensive overview will be reviewed, including studies using quantitative, qualitative, and mixed methods to examine auditory verbal hallucinations as experienced by both clinical populations and healthy voice-hearers. These studies were selected to demonstrate the ways in which clinical and non-clinical voice-hearers have been studied to date, as well as to highlight some of the similarities and differences in the experiences that each population had with auditory verbal hallucinations.

Sorrell et al. (2009) conducted a cross-sectional study that surveyed 32 clinical voice-hearers and 18 healthy voice-hearers using the Psychotic Symptoms Rating Scale (Haddock et al.,1999), the Voice and You questionnaire (Hayward, et al., 2008), the Beliefs About Voices Questionnaire – Revised (Chadwick et al., 2009), and the Beck Depression Inventory-II (Beck et al., 1996). The results found that healthy voice-hearers reported significantly less distress than did clinical voice-hearers (z = -4.58, p < .01, r = .65). They also perceived the voices to be less dominant (z = 4.61, p < .01, r = .65) and intrusive (z = -4.60, p < .01, r =.65) than the clinical group. This study highlighted the existence of healthy voice-hearers as well as their significantly lower amount of distress compared with the clinical population that experiences auditory verbal hallucinations. However, the self-report measures that participants completed provided a limited picture of personal experiences with the voices. This leaves a gap in the literature that qualitative studies could supplement through collecting personal accounts of both healthy and clinical voice-hearers. Additionally, this study used a small sample size, which could lead to insufficient power to detect a real effect even if it was present.

A phenomenological study by Taylor and Murray (2012) interviewed six people who identified as healthy voice-hearers who practiced mediumship and perceived their auditory verbal hallucinations as spirits. The interview transcripts were analyzed using Interpretive Phenomenological Analysis (Smith & Osborn, 2003); enabling the researchers to explore an individual's account of an experience while being actively involved with the data interpretations process (in other words, the researcher makes sense of how the interviewees make sense of their experiences).

The main themes resulting from this analysis used the term clairaudience to describe the voices that participants hear. Themes included the experience of the clairaudience, understanding clairauditory experiences and their meaning, and engaging with clairauditory and mediumistic experiences. For the first theme, Taylor and Murray (2012) found the participants' accounts of how they perceive the voices to be aligned with how clinical voice-hearers perceive voices. The second theme of understanding the experiences involved participants making meaning of the voices they hear and engaging with them in a manner they found to be personally beneficial. Finally, the third theme involved participants indicating that they have a choice of whether or not to engage with the voices that they hear. This reflected a difference between people who are considered healthy voice-hearers and clinical voice-hearers, because healthy voice-hearers report more control over the auditory verbal hallucinations they experience. Although this study may have been limited in its small, specific sample of people who identified as spiritual mediums, it provided refreshing insight into how making meaning of one's experiences could help them cope, and sometimes even actively engage, with voices they hear.

A mixed-methods study used questionnaire data to gather information on the phenomenology of auditory verbal hallucinations (Woods et al., 2015). People who experienced hearing voices ($N = 153$) were recruited to the study, including those with a psychiatric diagnosis ($n = 127$) and those without a diagnosis or mental health history ($n = 26$). Survey results showed that a greater percentage of clinical voice-hearers (39%) found the voices they heard to be negative and abusive than did healthy voice-hearers

(19%). Clinical participants also reported the voices being associated with fear (47%) than did healthy voice-hearers (12%). Nearly half of the non-clinical participants (46%) reported the voices being positive and even useful, compared with only 27% of the clinical sample reporting the same. The researchers used an inductive thematic analysis to code responses and used coded data to calculate descriptive statistics. However, there were no tests conducted to measure statistical significance of these findings.

Woods et al. (2015) claimed this research to be the largest collection of open-ended survey information on the phenomenology of voices. Although the sample did include people without a psychiatric diagnosis, this sample was small ($n = 26$) compared with the clinical sample also included ($n = 127$). Further, the sample of clinical voice-hearers was comprised of people with a non-psychotic disorder diagnosis (e.g., Borderline Personality Disorder, Major Depressive Disorder, Generalized Anxiety Disorder) in addition to those with a psychotic disorder (e.g., schizophrenia, schizoaffective disorder). This mixed sample raised questions about the extent to which healthy voice-hearers and people with psychosis may be compared, as these were not the only participants included in the study. However, this study's inclusion of a broad sample of people demonstrated the prevalence of auditory verbal hallucinations across multiple clinical and non-clinical presentations.

A review of the literature here provides a glimpse into the varied experiences of people who experience hearing voices, regardless of other mental health symptoms or diagnostic criteria they do or do not meet Although most of the clinical training that therapists receive in terms of psychotic symptoms focuses on people who meet diagnostic criteria for a psychotic disorder, the literature on healthy voice-hearers invites clinicians to take a fresh look at the experiences of people who hear voices and consider "thinking

outside the box" of pathology. With this new perspective in mind, therapeutic treatments

for people who experience psychotic symptoms at a clinical level will be reviewed for an

overview of which interventions are most frequently used by clinicians working with this

population.

Current Treatments for Psychosis

There is a lack of training as well as practical experience for clinicians working

with and understanding people with psychosis. Although clinicians from certain

disciplines (e.g., clinical psychology) may be trained in recognizing and treating positive

symptoms that are present in schizophrenia, Galderisi and others (2017) argued that there

is not much training associated with identification and treatment of the negative

symptoms present in schizophrenia. Additionally, there remains a gap in the training of

practitioners in counseling psychology programs around identifying symptoms of

psychosis and working with these clients. Further, there is a lack of consensus around

which interventions are most efficacious for treating people with psychosis. Although the

use of antipsychotic medication continues to be the most widely used and efficacious

treatment of symptoms of psychosis, researchers and clinicians are increasingly

advocating for the integration of psychopharmacological treatment with psychotherapy

(Kennedy & Xyrichis, 2017; Li et al., 2018; Menon et al., 2017; Newton-Howes &

Wood, 2011). A biopsychosocial approach to treatment is indicated to ensure best

outcomes (Lehman et al., 2010; NICE, 2010). Following a brief overview of medication

use in treating psychosis, multiple types of psychosocial interventions that are presently

used to treat people with psychosis are reviewed here. These approaches include some of the most frequently implemented treatments for people with psychosis, including cognitive-behavioral therapy for psychosis, mindfulness, peer support, and treatments for acute psychosis.

Antipsychotic Medication Treatments for Psychosis

Although a biopsychosocial approach that incorporates elements of medication, psychotherapy, and social support is indicated for best outcomes for people with psychosis (Lehman et al., 2010; NICE, 2010), sometimes medication is used as a standalone treatment approach. Antipsychotic medications are classified into two categories, first- and second-generation antipsychotics. First-generation antipsychotics are used to treat acute psychotic episodes, and sometimes as maintenance therapy for both schizophrenia and schizoaffective disorders (Yazici et al., 2017). This category of antipsychotics treats positive symptoms of psychosis (e.g., hallucinations, delusions), and can decrease the risk for a second episode of psychosis. Second-generation antipsychotics treat both positive and negative psychotic symptoms (e.g., withdrawal, ambivalence), and can reduce episodic relapse (Yazici et al., 2017). Although psychologists cannot currently prescribe psychotropic medications to patients in most US states, a review of several clinical studies conducted with patients who received antipsychotic medication as a standalone treatment by psychiatric prescribers is provided here.

A meta-analysis conducted by Leucht et al. (2012) used four databases to identify multiple studies ($N = 116$) that contained participants with schizophrenia being randomly assigned to a prescribed antipsychotic drug condition or a placebo condition ($N = 6,493$). The primary outcome that was used in the fixed effects model analysis was relapse. The researchers found that people in the drug treatment group had less relapse at one-year

follow-up compared to the placebo group (27% *vs.* 64%; *RR* = 0.40, 95% *CI* 0.33-0.49).
The findings also revealed that fewer patients in the treatment group were readmitted
than were those in the control group (10% *vs.* 26%, *RR* = 0.38, 95% *CI* 0.27-0.55). From
the meta-analysis, the authors concluded that patients receiving medication maintenance
treatment had significantly lower relapse rates than did the patients receiving no
medication.

Another study (Girgis et al., 2018) investigated the differences between first- and
second-generation antipsychotics (prescribed in the first psychotic episode) on the
outcomes of schizophrenia symptoms in the long term. The researchers open with a
review statement noting that acute-phase efficacy results show few differences between
classes of antipsychotic medications (e.g., Crespo-Facorro et al., 2006; Emsley, 1999). In
the presently reviewed study, Girgis et al. (2018) sought to learn about the comparative
effectiveness of antipsychotic drugs in first-episode psychosis and on long-term
outcomes. Participants (N = 160) in Beijing, China who were diagnosed with first-
episode schizophrenia (n = 76%) or schizophreniform disorder (n = 24%) were randomly
assigned to the first-generation medication (clozapine) group, or to the second-generation
medication (chlorpromazine) group. The researchers conducted efficacy assessments at
baseline, weekly for weeks 1-6, biweekly for weeks 6-12, at hospital discharge, and for
every three months following discharge for nine years. The data were analyzed using
general linear mixed modeling, and the primary outcome measured was remission status
of participants over the course of the observation period.

Participants in the clozapine group spent more time in remission during the first
year of observation and were faster to be in remission during the first year of treatment.

The average percentage of time that participants spent in each clinical state was identical across both treatment groups (e.g., remission [78%], intermediate [8%], and relapse [14%]). The main conclusions from the authors of this study are that no significant differences were found for the course of illness development between people taking first- or second-generation antipsychotics as their first medication for first-episode psychosis. Although the study design was in multiple ways ideal (e.g., longitudinal study, relatively large sample size, random assignment to groups), the authors made a declaration of intent acknowledging they received funding from multiple psychopharmacological companies, which may have biased their study design or interpretation of the findings. Additionally, this study only compared patients who were using medication and were not involved in psychosocial interventions. Keeping these limitations in mind, Girgis et al. (2018) still provided some insight into the potential efficacy of different antipsychotic medication classifications on people with first-episode psychosis, and the evidence supports antipsychotic medication management as an efficacious standalone treatment compared to no medication or other form of treatment. However, considering NICE's (2010) recommendation of adopting an integrative, biopsychosocial treatment approach for people with psychosis, I will return my discussion to a review of therapeutic treatment approaches to psychosis.

Cognitive-Behavioral Therapy for Psychosis

An increase in the implementation of Cognitive-behavioral therapy (CBT) in recent decades has led to the application of this approach to treating psychotic disorders. Cognitive-behavioral therapy for psychosis aims to assist people with psychosis in identifying, monitoring, and evaluating their assumptions, beliefs, and thoughts surrounding their psychotic experiences (Menon et al., 2017). A common therapeutic method in CBT for psychosis sessions involves the therapist helping the client identify and challenge their beliefs that may be maintaining their symptoms. Current evidence supports the efficacy and feasibility of CBT for psychosis in treating individuals with schizophrenia, but there is a lack of evidence to demonstrate its superiority compared with other treatments for people with psychosis (Menon et al., 2017).

A systematic review and meta-analysis by Newton-Howes and Wood (2011) examined whether CBT reduces psychopathology in individuals with schizophrenia more effectively than non-cognitive psychotherapies, as measured by a combination of measures including the PANSS, the Brief Psychiatric Rating Scale, the Scale for the Assessment of Negative Symptoms, and the Perceptual Aberration Scale. This meta-analysis searched three databases and included nine placebo controlled randomized controlled trials (RCTs) that met all inclusion criteria, involving 602 patients in total. Data were combined using a random effect model. No significant difference was found in symptom reduction between patients being treated with CBT and those receiving different treatment ($MD = 0.04$, $CI = -0.29 - .036$).

A meta-analysis by Zimmermann et al. (2005) examined the efficacy of CBT for psychosis in the treatment of positive symptoms of schizophrenia spectrum disorders. Fourteen studies totaling 1,484 participants were used in the meta-analysis. A small to moderate mean effect size (ES) across all studies was found; the fixed effect model (FEM) mean weighted ES was 0.35 (95% CI: $0.23 - 0.47$), and the random effect model (REM) mean weighted ES was 0.37 (95% CI: $0.23 - 0.52$). This finding suggested that a typical participant in the CBT group showed greater improvements than more than 64%

of the control group; and that CBT increased the rate of reducing positive symptoms from 59% to 41%. These results across the examined studies provided support for the general conclusion that CBT is a promising approach for treating positive symptoms in clients with schizophrenia. Additionally, the therapeutic effects persisted at follow-up, suggesting that CBT has long-term utility. However, a two-way analysis of variance (ANOVA) was conducted using unbiased ES as a dependent variable and patient status (chronic vs. acute) and control treatment format (non-specific, treatment as usual, waiting-list) as independent variables. No significant group effects (patient status: F (1, 16) = 1.08, $p > .05$; control treatment format: F (2, 15) = .30, $p > .05$) or interaction effects (F (2, 15) = .76, $p > .05$) were found. This finding demonstrated that there were not significant differences between comparison groups (non-specific interventions and/or supportive therapy) and CBT groups.

Another meta-analysis conducted by Kennedy and Xyrichis (2017) examined the evidence available for using CBT compared to non-specialized therapy with people with schizophrenia, specifically regarding their reports of auditory hallucinations, as measured by The Positive and Negative Syndrome Scale (PANSS; Kay et al., 1987). Only two RCTs met the inclusion criteria for this analysis (Penn et al., 2009; Shawyer et al., 2012), with a combined sample size of 105 participants. RCTs involve random assignment to experiment or control groups, intervention for the experimental group, and baseline equivalence for groups in the analytic sample (Kabisch et al. 2011) and are widely considered the "gold standard" of research design (Chambless & Hollon, 1998). The pooled analysis found no statistically significant difference in terms of reducing positive symptoms between CBT and non-specialized therapy groups (MD = -0.86, CI = -2.38 -

.065, $p = 0.26$). While the authors acknowledged the limitation of a small sample size and limited number of studies, they concluded that there was no significant difference between the two forms of therapy in terms of auditory hallucinations or other positive symptoms. Several of the RCTs that were included in this meta-analysis are reviewed in detail below and highlight key findings from using CBT for people who experience auditory verbal hallucinations.

An RCT by Penn and colleagues (2009) compared group CBT with enhanced supportive therapy for people with auditory verbal hallucinations. This study included sixty-five participants with diagnoses of schizophrenia spectrum disorders and persistent hallucinations. Participants were randomly assigned to group CBT ($n = 32$) or enhanced group supportive therapy ($n = 33$). Participants who received group CBT did not report a reduction in voice distress or intensity, whereas those in the supportive group did experience this reduction. However, those in the CBT condition reported lower general symptom scores on the PANSS through twelve-month follow-up ($F (1, 58) = 5.74, p = .02, d = -.63$) compared with supportive therapy group participants. Outcomes continued to improve through 12-month follow-up in both therapy groups. The authors acknowledged limitations in their study in terms of a small sample size ($N = 65$) which allowed for only moderate to large differences between the two groups They concluded that both CBT and supportive treatment had some beneficial outcomes for people with psychosis, but on different outcomes.

Another RCT examined acceptance-based CBT for people with psychotic disorders who experiences auditory verbal hallucinations that give verbal commands (Shawyer et al., 2012). Forty-three participants who experienced command hallucinations received random assignment to an acceptance-based CBT treatment group ($n = 21$) or a control group of non-specialized therapy ($n = 22$), then followed up with six months after termination. The study found that participants in the acceptance-based CBT group reported greater improvement in reducing command hallucinations, but there was no significant difference between this and the non-CBT group on primary and secondary outcome measures in terms of participants' confidence in resisting harmful commands (F (1, 35) = 0.05, $p = .82$). However, compared with waitlist participants ($n = 17$), participants in both treatment groups combined showed significant improvement in confidence in coping with commands and quality of life. The authors concluded that although the sample size for this study is small ($N = 43$), the results suggested that CBT appeared to be effective for people with psychosis compared with no treatment but was not superior to supportive treatment in terms of outcome measures. This finding appeared to be present across multiple original studies and meta-analyses of the literature, as detailed in this section. Next, the use of mindfulness interventions for treatment of psychosis will be detailed.

Mindfulness Interventions for Psychosis

Another type of intervention that has been applied to work with people with psychosis incorporates mindfulness. Specific types of these interventions that are reviewed in a systematic review by Aust and Bradshaw (2017) include: (a) Acceptance and Commitment Therapy (Hayes et al., 1999), (b) Acceptance-Based Cognitive Behavioral Therapy (Braehler et al., 2013), (c)Mindfulness-Based Cognitive Therapy (Segal et al., 2002), (d) Mindfulness-Based Psychoeducation Programme (Chien & Lee, 2013), (e) Mindfulness Intervention for Rehabilitation and Recovery in Schizophrenia

(Davis et al., 2015), (f) Person-Based Cognitive Therapy (Chadwick et al., 2009), (g) and self-help, Internet-based mindfulness interventions (Moritz et al., 2015). Mindfulness interventions for psychosis (mindfulness interventions for psychosis) may vary in their specific techniques, but share the common goal of negative emotion regulation through increasing a person's willingness to embrace the experience of the present moment (Khoury et al., 2013). There is some debate surrounding the use of mindfulness interventions with this population because meditation-induced psychosis has been documented in several studies (Shonin et al., 2014).

However, in their review, Aust and Bradshaw (2017) noted important methodological limitations for the studies that called this into question. For the literature synthesis, thirteen studies detailing eleven RCTs using mindfulness interventions for psychosis met inclusion criteria. The authors found mindfulness interventions for psychosis to be feasible options for people with psychosis. However, they discovered there to be varying quality to the RCTs that they analyzed, so they cautioned that the evidence was therefore stronger for some specific mindfulness interventions for psychosis compared with others (for example, Mindfulness-based Psychoeducation Programme had higher-quality evidence for its effectiveness than Mindfulness Intervention for Recovery and Rehabilitation in Schizophrenia). Through their review, the authors found no ill effects in any of the studies. Thus, they concluded that mindfulness interventions can be safely administered if they are carefully adapted to the special needs of individuals with psychosis. Aust and Bradshaw (2017) also cautioned that a universal consensus for how mindfulness is defined does not exist, suggesting a need for future agreement on how to conceptualize this before making general conclusions about its efficacy for people with psychosis.

An RCT conducted by Chadwick et al. (2009) compared a group-based mindfulness intervention ($n = 9$) with a waitlisted control group ($n = 6$) for people with psychosis. They found that participants in the mindfulness intervention group reported significant improvements in mindfulness of distressing thoughts and images, per the Southampton Mindfulness Questionnaire (95% *CI* [0.6,16.0], $p < .05$), which measures the extent to which respondents respond mindfully to distressing stimuli. The authors acknowledged limitations in their study in terms of very small sample size and limited statistical power. However, this study provided some indication that mindfulness-based interventions may be feasible for people with psychosis and associated with some positive outcomes.

Another RCT was conducted by Langer et al. (2012). This study compared participants receiving mindfulness-based cognitive therapy ($n = 7$) with a waitlisted control group ($n = 11$). After treatment, all participants completed several outcome measures, including the Southampton Mindfulness Questionnaire. The study found that the participants in the mindfulness-based CBT intervention were better able to respond mindfully to internal events that were stressful than those who received no treatment. However, there were multiple methodological weaknesses in this study. Langer et al. (2012) used a very small sample that was also unequally distributed between groups due to attrition. Additionally, the control group did not receive any type of treatment, which limited this study to comparing some type of treatment to no treatment.

A pilot RCT by Lopez-Navarro et al. (2015) examined the effectiveness of group mindfulness-based intervention in patients with SMI. The mindfulness intervention group ($n = 22$) received weekly mindfulness group therapy in addition to integrated rehabilitation treatment, which included pharmacotherapy and weekly CBT that focused on symptom management. The control group ($n = 22$) only received integrated rehabilitation treatment without the mindfulness intervention. Both groups of participants received their respective interventions over the course of 26 weeks and completed the PANSS and the WHOQOL-BREF at baseline and post-intervention. Through ANOVA analysis, the researchers found that participants in the group that included mindfulness intervention indicated improved quality of life (e.g. increased self-esteem, positive feelings, body image, and reduced frequency of negative feelings). This study used a sample that was comprised of participants with SMI, only 89% of which were diagnosed with schizophrenia, and was limited to a single site of data collection (a public community rehabilitation center). Additionally, Lopez-Navarro et al. (2015) only conducted a pilot study and indicated the study could be expanded to a full clinical trial including longitudinal data. Despite some limitations, this study showed the additive factor of mindfulness interventions compared with CBT and pharmacotherapy alone.

Using mindfulness-based interventions is one approach that clinicians may consider when working with people with psychosis. Incorporating mindfulness into therapy may help clients have more control over their distressing thoughts and learn how to remain grounded in the present moment and aware of their experiences. However, the extent of evidence showing the efficacy for these interventions as the primary form of treatment is relatively weak, due to limited samples and lack of rigor across multiple studies. To continue the discussion on empirically supported treatments for psychosis, the peer support approach will be reviewed next.

Peer Support Treatments for Psychosis

Another therapeutic approach that is sometimes used with people with psychosis is incorporating peer support into treatment. Peer support in a mental health setting is generally defined by a peer with personal mental health experience providing emotional, appraisal, and informational assistance to others experiencing similar mental health difficulties (Chien et al., 2019). An underlying assumption of the peer support approach is that people who have had similar experiences to clients currently in treatment are considered more equal in the therapeutic relationship than are clients and professional therapists (Dennis, 2003). Some of the benefits as well as limitations of this approach will be discussed below through a review of literature on peer support treatments for people with psychosis. Some of the effects of peer-supported interventions compared with non-peer interventions were explored in a systematic review by Chien et al. (2019), which will be detailed below.

Chien et al. (2019) completed a systematic review that consisted of 13 qualitative and 12 quantitative studies that compared peer support treatments to other psychosocial interventions led by clinicians. The primary outcomes that were measured by the studies included hospital admission and duration of time hospitalized, relapse, clinically significant improvement in global state, and quality of life. There were no significant differences found between peer-supported and clinican-directed treatment in terms of emergency service use and hospital admissions, but Chien et al. (2019) acknowledge that limited data were present across studies to measure this outcome (*RR* 0.44, 95% *CI* 0.11

to 1.75) (Reynolds, 2004). This systematic review also found limited data across studies to measure relapse and global state between groups. The closest measurement of global state were endpoint measurements on global state scales; one study found no difference between peer support and clinician-led treatment at both medium and long term follow-up as measured by the VR-12 (*MD* -0.02, 95% *CI* -3.96 to 3.92) (Eisen, 2012), and another study found a favorable score difference for peer support at medium term follow-up, but a favorable score difference for clinician-led care at long-term follow-up (Mahlke et al., 2017). Finally, Chien et al. (2019) reviewed quality of life outcomes across studies, as measured by scale scores for quality of life (including components such as overall quality of life, mental health, physical health, social functioning, and living arrangements). Overall, Chien et al. (2019) found no significant difference in quality of life subscale scores. This systematic review found some limited support for peer support interventions (e.g., improvements in global scale measures at medium term follow-up, Mahlke et al., 2017) and some limited support for clinician-led standard care (e.g., improvements in global scale measures at long term follow-up, Mahlke et al., 2017), but overall did not find significant differences between treatments.

Next, some specific studies from the systematic review by Chien et al. (2019) will be detailed to highlight some of the different ways that peer support interventions for psychosis have been studied for efficacy across multiple outcomes. The first of these studies is a randomized controlled trial by Castelein et al. (2008) that investigated the effects of a guided peer support group for people with psychosis. Across multiple sites, the researchers compared patients with a psychotic disorder in the peer support group (*n* = 56) with patients with a psychotic disorder in the standard care control condition (*n* =

50) on outcomes including social support, self-efficacy, and quality of life. The peer support group involved sixteen sessions of 90-minute groups, biweekly over the course of eight months. Patients took self-report measures (e.g., Social Support List, Mental Health Confidence Scale, Rosenberg scale, and WHO Quality of Life Brief) at baseline and at eight-month follow-up. The researchers used general linear model analyses to examine changes in self-report scores from baseline to follow-up between groups. They found mixed results; patients in the peer support group reported higher increases compared to the control group in social support (*RR* 1.85, 95% *CI* 1.14 to 3.00) as well as a modest but insignificant increases in self-efficacy (*MD* 2.70, 95% *CI* -2.40 to 7.80) and quality of life (*MD* 1.70, 95% *CI* -2.32 to 5.72). However, there were no differences between groups on other outcomes, including relationships outside of the mental health environment and self-esteem (*MD* 0.50, 95% *CI* -1.22 to 2.22).

Another RCT, conducted by Cook et al. (2012) tested the efficacy of a peer-led mental illness intervention for patients with schizophrenia against a control group across multiple outcomes. Patients of mental health services (*N* = 428) from eight different community mental health settings in rural Tennessee were recruited through their therapists, peer referral, newspaper advertisement, and snowball sampling, and were randomly assigned to a peer intervention (*n* = 212) or standard care control (*n* = 216) group. The peer support intervention and standard care were delivered to their respective participants once a week for eight weeks, and participants took self-report measures at baseline as well as two time points (medium and long term) following the study. Cook et al. (2012) found a significant decrease in depressive symptoms measured by the Brief Symptom Inventory at medium-term follow up for patients in the peer support group

(*MD* -0.13, 95% *CI* -0.25 to -0.01), but no difference between groups at long-term follow-up (*MD* 0.00, 95% *CI* -0.11 to 0.11). They also found that participants receiving peer support reported significantly higher quality of life as measured by the WHO Quality of Life Brief at long-term follow-up compared with the standard care group (*MD* 0.70, 95% *CI* 0.15 to 1.25). Additionally, patients in the peer support group reported more improved confidence than the control group at the end of treatment (*MD* 1.90, 95% *CI* 0.61 to 3.19), as measured by the Recovery Assessment Scale.

Although there is evidence demonstrating the potential efficacy of several types of treatment (particularly, CBT, mindfulness interventions, and peer support interventions, as outlined here) for use with people with psychosis, it appears that there is not one type of psychotherapy that is clearly more effective than others. Multiple studies acknowledge this limitation in their findings, and attribute some of the success of each treatment approach to common factors, including client and therapist characteristics, adherence to the theory of a treatment model, and the therapeutic alliance between the client and therapist (Wampold & Imel, 2015). Because these common factors are present across different types of interventions, there is opportunity for more in-depth study on how these factors may contribute to treatment outcomes, and not be exclusive to CBT, mindfulness, or peer support interventions for psychosis.

Treatments for Acute Psychosis

Many of the treatment approaches that have been reviewed so far have focused on interventions that are best indicated for people who meet criteria for the mild to moderate range of schizophrenia and for people who have been stabilized and are not experiencing an acute psychotic episode. However, people who are experiencing acute or brief psychosis can benefit from different approaches.

A meta-analysis by Paterson et al. (2018) drew information from 512 studies retrieved from online databases, reference lists, and reviews to learn about the benefit of therapy for patients in acute inpatient mental health care. After applying exclusion criteria, the authors narrowed their data pool to include 20 RCT trial studies that compared multiple psychotherapy interventions including CBT ($n = 11$), MCT ($n = 3$), ACT ($n = 2$), DBT ($n = 1$), eye-movement desensitization and reprocessing ($n = 1$), interpersonal psychotherapy ($n = 1$), and social skills training ($n = 1$) to "treatment as usual" ($n = 13$), treatment as usual plus a comparator intervention ($n = 3$), psychoeducation ($n = 2$), cognitive remediation ($n =1$), and supportive counseling ($n = 1$). Paterson and colleagues (2018) found that psychological therapy was associated with a small-to-medium benefit over comparators on all outcomes (SMD -0.39; CI -0.64 to -0.14; $p = .00$). The primary outcomes were psychotic symptoms as measured by pre- and post-test scores on the PANSS (Kay et al., 1987), and secondary outcomes included self-reported emotional distress and risk of readmission. No significant differences were found among types of therapy, indicating that any of the utilized approaches were more effective in treating brief psychosis than the comparators. The researchers (Paterson et al., 2018) acknowledged that their meta-analysis only focused on studies that used directive approaches (e.g., CBT, DBT, ACT) instead of non-directive approaches (e.g., person-centered therapy), but indicated that this analysis reflects the approaches that are typically used in acute inpatient settings for this population. They conclude that these directive approaches can be beneficial to clients experiencing acute psychosis, but also indicate that the most important factor in these treatments is giving clients the

opportunity to spend time with a trained therapist.

The present study focuses on people who may demonstrate symptoms that align

with the mild range of psychosis, and those who do not consider the voices they hear to

be symptoms at all. It is important to acknowledge the distinction between people who

experience none, mild, or moderate symptoms or distress and those who experience their

symptoms as severe.

Meaning-Making

There is a growing interest in understanding the role of the therapist in helping

people with psychosis make sense of their experiences in a way that increases their sense

of agency and self-worth, provides hope for the future, and allows for the processing of

distress (Dilks et al., 2012). Meaning-making processes are shaped through ongoing

interactions that a person has in various social and institutional contexts, as well as by the

individual's personal history (Roe & Davidson, 2005). Helping people with psychosis

make meaning of their experiences is illustrated through several studies described here,

ranging from a theoretical framework design to a grounded theory analysis. Empirical

studies using quantitative methods to examine meaning-making in people with psychosis

populations have not been identified, suggesting there is a lack of literature presently

available on this topic, particularly a lack of studies employing rigorous methodology.

Additionally, the present literature on using meaning-making approaches with people

with psychosis is sparse, indicating a need for more research in this area.

Roe et al. (2006) outlined the design of a clinically useful framework for helping

people cope with psychotic experiences. They discussed the benefits of proactive coping, in which individuals shift from reacting to actively making meaning of events and viewing themselves as meaning-making beings. Acceptance, flexible reappraisal, and ultimately, a self that can admit suffering and incorporate the universal human experience of pain and suffering into one's life are pieces of a person's experiences when they are proactively coping. An example of proactive coping provided by Roe et al. (2006) was a person with psychosis who initiated looking for a job and began to make meaning through productive, engaging work. They suggested that when working with people with psychosis, the clinician's role in facilitating proactive coping would not just focus on psychoeducation or symptom management, but also on facilitating the growth of one's self as a personal meaning maker. The aim of facilitating this growth is for the client to arrive at a place where they feel they are attuned to the world and able to interact with it in a sense of meaningful identity and existence in the world (Roe et al., 2006).

In a grounded theory analysis of therapy and recovery processes in people with psychosis, Dilks et al. (2012) addressed the question of how a therapist can both respect a client's personal meaning-making and also introduce a different perspective, assuming the client is using problematic meaning-making. In their grounded theory analysis, the researchers analyzed taped therapy sessions involving six pairs of psychologists and clients with psychosis, as well as conducted 23 interviews from therapy sample participants. Several grounded theory categories emerged from the data. One such category was classified as building a bridge to observational perspectives (defining the central process in psychological therapy in psychosis). This involved an ongoing conversation between therapist and client in taking different perspectives. Through this, the client was able to process emotion and open up to new possibilities for thought, feeling, and action. A main goal associated with this category is to enable the client to move towards functioning in the social world. More themes related to bridge-building included: (a) working to maintain observational perspectives, (b) defining the subcomponents of working to maintain observational perspectives, (c) managing emotion, and (d) doing relationship (a reciprocal process of psychologist and client working together to develop a confiding, respectful relationship). A conclusion from Dilks et al. (2012) is that a common theme is that it is helpful for the clinician to both assist the person experiencing psychosis to manage emotional intensity at a tolerable level and to assist them in opening up new ways of thinking about their experience.

Helping clients to make meaning of their psychotic experiences can help to empower individuals by allowing them to take an active role in the understanding of their experiences as well as in their treatment. As discussed in the earlier section on healthy voice-hearers, there are individuals who experience hearing voices and have the ability to cope, and sometimes even meaningfully engage with these experiences. Learning more from people who are classified as healthy voice-hearers can provide additional insight into how these individuals use some of their strengths to actively cope with these experiences without decreasing functioning across multiple areas of life. Understanding these experiences from a critical theory framework can help clinicians empower clients to transcend the barriers of stigma and misunderstanding and make meaning of their experiences.

A Shift to Positive Psychotherapy

Many of the present treatments for people with psychosis operate from a deficit-based perspective. That is, they seek to reduce or remove psychotic symptoms and help clients improve their social and occupational functioning. Positive psychology emerged as a response to the medical model's focus of classifying and pathologizing people based on their presenting symptoms. Positive psychology aims to increase well-being through helping people understand and build positive emotions, gratification, and meaning (Seligman et al., 2004). It employs a strengths-based perspective that is a multimodal endeavor, exploring both strengths and weaknesses in clients (Rashid & Ostermann, 2009). A sole focus on a client's deficits reinforces a fundamental negative bias and runs the risk of reducing the person to a diagnostic label. Positive psychology has experienced skepticism from some researchers and clinicians. Lazarus (2003) criticized the positive psychology movement as focusing too narrowly on positive emotions and denying the reality that some clients experience debilitating symptoms that negatively impact their functioning. Despite some critiques of positive psychology, the positive psychology movement does not call for an abandonment of a client's negative experiences and distress. Rather, Martin Seligman, one of the founding clinicians who spurred the positive psychology movement, argued for a shift towards psychology being just as concerned with what is right as is with what is wrong with people (Seligman et al., 2004; Seligman & Pawelski, 2003). Positive psychology extends beyond the study of how we feel and includes strengths, virtues, and meaning, not just happy feelings. Seligman and other proponents of positive psychology envisioned a balanced psychology that integrates research on positive states and traits with research on suffering and pathology. They predicted that eventually, there will be no distinct separation between "psychology as usual" and positive psychology; elements of positive psychology will be blended into mainstream psychology and an inseparable piece of theory and treatment. Another criticism by Lazarus (2003) was that positive psychology relates mostly to affluent, middle-aged white men, largely because many of its founders and early proponents fit this demographic picture. Seligman responded to this critique, acknowledging the lack of diversity in the movement's founders, but insisting strengths and virtues can be identified that are valued regardless of cultural variables (Seligman & Pawelski, 2003).

Other researchers have identified areas where positive psychology is lacking in terms of diversity and representation. Rao and Donaldson (2015) examined these biases of the field through conducting a systematic review of positive psychology literature spanning seventeen years (N = 1,628 English-language articles from five databases, from the years 1998-2014). The content analysis found that gender discrepancies; women are overrepresented as participants in studies (n = 60.2% in aggregate) but underrepresented in terms of first authorship of the conducted studies (n = 43%). This finding supports critics' claims that the bulk of the positive psychology literature comes from male researchers and clinicians. Additionally, Rao and Donaldson (2015) discovered a lack of diversity in the samples across studies; participants were predominantly white, and there was sparse discussion on race, ethnicity, or the role of intersecting identities in clients' lives. Implications from this systematic review include a need for expanding positive psychology research to include (and even focus on) the role of clients' intersecting identities in their lived experiences. Although Seligman may have been ambitious in his attempt to locate universal commonalities shared by all people, he risked neglecting key multicultural identity considerations that contribute to individuals' unique experiences. Additionally, the research that has followed Seligman's pioneering work has continued to neglect these key variables. This is one criticism to keep in mind when advocating for and using positive psychology-informed approaches with clients.

Wood and Tarrier (2010) provided an argument for an integrated positive clinical approach in their critical review of both the positive psychology movement and clinical psychology. They provided some critique towards the field of clinical psychology; arguing that it focuses primarily on the negative aspects of patients and their illnesses. They argued that positive psychology in its current state encourages practitioners to solely focus on positive aspects of the people they work with. Another criticism they provided is that positive psychology is often considered to be a new movement; however, it is not a new idea. It can be argued that positive psychology has its roots in the humanistic movement, perhaps beginning with Maslow (1970) and the outline for human potential that is provided in his hierarchy of needs and his suggestion that people can reach their full potential through self-actualization. Credit is also given to the field of counseling psychology for rejecting the deficit orientation and focusing on strengths. Another criticism is that positive psychology fails to integrate both the positive and negative. Inadequate evaluation of interventions is also noted, citing a lack of literature on the effectiveness of positive psychotherapy interventions. Finally, after acknowledging these criticisms, the authors called for a reorientation of clinical psychology that equally balances positive and negative functioning when predicting, understanding, and treating distress. It is suggested that this be accomplished through re-conceptualizing the relationship between positive and negative well-being, rigorous evaluation of positive interventions, and reconsidering the role of clinical psychologists as targeting only distress rather than improving well-being.

Since Wood and Tarrier (2010) wrote about the differences between clinical and positive psychology and called for a blending of the two areas, there have been several efforts to accomplish this aim. In 2017, Siddaway et al. tested two key predictions of positive clinical psychology, originally proposed by an earlier work of Wood and Tarrier (2010). These predictions were that many mental health problems can be understood as one end of a continuum (ranging from disorder to well-being), and that reducing psychiatric symptoms can provide an equal decrease in the risk for other psychiatric variables, regardless of where the person is on the continuum. Siddaway et al. (2017) used the Center for Epidemiologic Studies-Depression (CES-D) with a sample of 4,138 adolescents and adults (ages 13-21) who took part in a five-year longitudinal health survey study in a content factor analysis. The researchers found that depression can be conceptualized along a continuum, based on survey responses that measure symptom severity based on a combination of both depressive and well-being experiences. They also found that baseline levels on the depression/well-being continuum have a near-linear relationship with the outcome variables measured at baseline and one and two years later.

The study by Siddaway et al. (2017) has important implications for the inclusion of positive psychology in clinical practice, particularly for practitioners with clinical psychology backgrounds. Viewing mental health symptoms as a continuum from well-being to disorder may reduce diagnostic stigma, as everyone falls somewhere on the continuum. Further, practitioners can consider shifting their treatment focus from only reducing mental health symptoms to increasing well-being. This study also provides an example of ways that clinical psychology can integrate core concepts of positive psychology into its work; rather than completely abandon the deficit model, deficits may be viewed in a dual way alongside well-being and positive attributes. However, most of the literature that encourages a positive clinical psychology is composed by the same group of authors (e.g., Siddaway et al., 2017; Wood & Johnson, 2016; Wood & Tarrier, 2010) and provides more speculation and suggestion than it does evidence for a positive clinical psychology approach. Further, there is a lack of research on understanding people with psychosis through a positive clinical lens.

As noted in the introduction section of this paper, there is considerable overlap between counseling psychology and positive psychology in terms of core principles (APA, 1999; Gelso & Fretz, 2001; Savickas, 2003). This notion was empirically tested through a content analysis on counseling psychology literature over the last 50 years by Lopez et al. (2006). The researchers selected a random sample of 20% (N = 1,135) of the articles published in the Journal of Counseling Psychology, the Journal of Career Assessment, and the Journal of Multicultural Counseling and Development. Results found that 29% of articles randomly selected had a positive focus. The analysis of rating consistency across coders showed that the coders shared sufficient consensus ($k = .94$) in agreeing upon the articles that met content analysis criteria for positive content. A key conclusion from Lopez and colleagues (2006) about their study is that counseling psychology scholarship has promoted an increased understanding of positives in psychology and can continue to benefit from continuing to build on this connection. Some of the interventions that are guided by positive psychology are discussed next, in terms of working with clients that both do and do not meet criteria for a psychotic disorder.

Positive Psychology Interventions

The following section provides a review of several types of intervention guided by positive psychology that may be implemented by clinicians. As previously mentioned, researchers should maintain awareness of some limitations of the existing literature on the positive psychology approach, keeping in mind that since many interventions were normed on a homogenous sample, they may not be applicable to a wide range of diverse clients. With this attentive eye to diversity in mind, several interventions from a positive psychology framework are explored in some detail below.

A meta-analysis by Bolier et al. (2013) reviewed the effectiveness of positive psychology interventions for the general public as well as individuals with specific psychosocial problems. The researchers took a different approach to their meta-analysis by studying positive psychotherapy interventions in not only people with psychosocial problems, but the general population as well. The outcome measures selected were subjective well-being, psychological well-being, and depressive symptoms. The meta-analysis used a systematic literature search using PsychInfo, PubMed, and the Cochrane Central Register of Controlled Trials, from 1998 (the beginning of the positive psychology movement) to November 2012. Forty articles describing 39 studies were included.

Results found that positive psychotherapy interventions were effective for all three outcomes as post-test effects. A moderate, significant effect size was observed for subjective well-being (Cohen's $d = 0.34$, 95% CI [0.22, 0.45], $p < .01$), and a small but significant effect sizes were found for psychological well-being (Cohen's $d = 0.20$, 95% CI [0.09, 0.30], $p <.01$), and depression (Cohen's $d = 0.23$, 95% CI [0.09, 0.38], $p <.01$).

Ten of the included studies examined follow-up effects from three to six months post-treatment. Small but significant effects were found in the treatment group in terms of subjective well-being (Cohen's $d = 0.22$, 95% CI [0.05, 0.38], $p < .01$) and for psychological well-being (Cohen's $d = .016$, 95% CI [0.02, 0.30], $p = .03$) in these studies. However, the effect was not significant for depression at follow-up (Cohen's $d = 0.17$, 95% CI [-0.06, 0.39], $p = .15$). An overall conclusion of this study was that positive psychotherapy interventions could be effective in enhancing subjective and psychological well-being and may help reduce depressive symptoms. The unique contributions made to the existing literature with this meta-analysis included using only RCTs, accounting for the methodological quality of primary studies, including the most recent studies, analyzing both post-test effects and long-term effects at follow-up, and applying clear inclusion criteria for the type of interventions as well as the study design.

One RCT reviewed in Boiler's (2013) meta-analysis examined a positive psychology intervention of writing, talking, and thinking about significant life events by Lyubomirsky et al. (2006). As the authors reviewed the prior literature, they noted that writing about positive emotions associated with a traumatic event is associated with lower heart rate (Hughes et al., 1994) and better immune functioning (Fredrickson & Levenson, 1998), speculating that focusing on positive emotions provides psychological resilience to face health threats. In Lyubomirsky and colleagues' (2006) study, they randomly assigned 111 undergraduate students to an intervention group: writing (independently on paper), talking (to a tape recorder), or thinking (independently) about a significant positive life event, or to the control group. Baseline and follow-up (four weeks post-test) measures were provided to all participants, including the Satisfaction with Life

Scale (Diener et al., 1985) which measures life satisfaction, the Positive and Negative Affect Schedule (Watson et al., 1988), measuring affect, the Medical Outcomes Study (Stewart et al.,1988) which measures general health, and the Symptom Checklist (Sherbourne et al., 1992), which measures common health problems.

The researchers found that participants in all three intervention groups (writing, talking, and thinking) scored higher post-test on all measures than did the control group. They additionally found that students who talked or wrote about their experiences showed more improvement from baseline to follow-up in terms of positive affect and overall health, whereas students in the thinking group showed greater improvement in life satisfaction. This study demonstrated the benefits from recalling and processing positive events on both mental and physical health, providing additional support to the literature about the role of focusing on the positive to build resilience. The sample used in this study was limited due to convenience sampling and was conducted on individuals who reported no mental health diagnosis, potentially limiting the generalizability of the results to clinical populations, specifically those who meet criteria for SMI.

Some of the studies included in Bolier's (2013) meta-analysis focused on a sample of people with psychosis. One such RCT that examined the effectiveness of one type of positive psychotherapy intervention with people with psychosis was conducted by Schrank et al. (2016). This study used a positive psychotherapy intervention referred to as WELLFOCUS positive psychotherapy, which consists of four target areas that include increasing positive experiences, amplifying strengths, fostering positive relationships, and creating self-narratives that are more meaningful. Participants ($N = 94$) were a convenience sample of people between 18-65 years of age with a primary diagnosis of psychosis who were actively participating in mental health services. Patients were randomized in blocks to receive either treatment as usual, or WELLFOCUS positive psychotherapy in addition to treatment as usual, administered as an 11-week group intervention. An ANCOVA revealed significant effects on psychotic symptoms ($p = 0.006$, ES = 0.42) and depression ($p = 0.03$, ES = 0.38) for the treatment group using the Warwick-Edinburgh Mental Well-Being Scale, the primary outcome scale as a measure. According to another measure, the Positive Psychotherapy Inventory, there were significant positive effects for well-being on people receiving WELLFOCUS positive psychotherapy ($p = 0.02$, ES = 0.30). Findings from this study suggested that incorporating elements of positive psychotherapy into treatment may have produced more positive outcomes than treatment as usual. The study also demonstrated the feasibility of implementing positive psychotherapy in a group intervention setting.

A pilot study examining a positive psychotherapy intervention specifically for people with psychosis was detailed in an article by Meyer et al. (2012). Here, the researchers adapted a group positive psychotherapy known as positive living for use with people with schizophrenia. These adaptations included addressing cognitive impairments, adding a positive goal to help people connect the group activities to their personal experiences, and adding a mindfulness exercise. The sample was comprised of sixteen people between the ages of 18-60 with a diagnosis of schizophrenia or schizoaffective disorder. All participants received the positive living intervention. Although there was no control group for comparison, Meyer et al. (2012) used a method consistent with the stepwise process of developing manualized treatment, including treatment conceptualization, treatment standardization, and pilot testing.

Repeated-measures ANOVAs were conducted to measure changes in participants' psychological well-being, symptoms, and social functioning from baseline to post-intervention, as well as at three-month follow-up. The results indicated that participants showed significant improvements in terms of well-being and symptom reduction from baseline (Well-being: $M = 201.6$, $SD = 34.46$; Symptoms: $M = 1.27$, $SD = 0.66$) to both post-intervention (Well-being: $M = 226.3$, $SD = 34.46$, $F = 11.77$; Symptoms: $M = 0.84$, $SD = 0.58$, $F = 6.51$) and three-month follow-up (Well-being: $M = 226.0$, $SD = 27.10$, $F = 7.37$; Symptoms: $M = 0.77$, $SD = 0.42$, $F = 12.17$). Participants showed small but insignificant improvements in social functioning from baseline ($M = 122.7$, $SD = 22.02$) to post-intervention ($M = 131.8$, $SD = 18.77$, $F = 4.15$) and three-month follow-up ($M = 130.3$, $SD = 25.66$, $F = 2.48$). Although this pilot study has design limitations of being a pre- and post-intervention study with no control group, it provided support for the feasibility of adapting positive psychotherapy interventions to people with psychosis, as well as support for the effectiveness of a positive psychotherapy intervention program in improving some patient outcomes.

In addition to using positive psychotherapy interventions to treat people who have already developed symptoms of psychosis, strengths-based interventions may be used with people who are at a clinically high risk for the development of psychosis. Drvaric et al. (2015) conducted a literature review that attempted to characterize the evidence base that related to psychosocial interventions that were oriented toward improving well-being and life satisfaction with a population at risk for psychosis. The population addressed by these studies was individuals who were identified as being at clinically high risk for psychosis development. Well-being was selected as an outcome of interest due to the literature neglecting to address this variable. The majority of studies reviewed focused on defining recovery in terms of symptom reduction. The authors searched through four databases for articles, narrowing their sample to eleven RCTs that used psychosocial interventions for clinically high-risk individuals.

Ultimately, Drvaric et al. (2015) made an argument for protective factors (such as well-being and resilience) as a key component of psychosocial interventions for people at clinically high risk for psychosis. Positive psychotherapy and its strengths-based approach was recommended as a treatment option, particularly for high-risk youth. They called it a resilience-boosting approach based on principles of building strengths, in contrast to the traditional approach of fixing something that is viewed as "broken" or "wrong." Through their analysis of the existing literature, the authors concluded that positive psychotherapy has shown effectiveness in both nonclinical and clinical populations and requires additional RCTs to determine if this type of therapy is effective with individuals at clinically high risk for psychosis development. They recommended positive psychotherapy be used as a complement to already well-established therapeutic approaches for the time being, or potentially as an alternative to other treatments.

Another approach to conceptualizing and working with people with psychosis that shares overlap with positive psychology is the recovery model. Rather than focusing on fully removing symptoms, this approach emphasizes resilience and a sense of control over one's life (Jacob, 2015). Adopting a recovery-oriented approach allows clinicians to view clients in a holistic way and views recovery as a journey rather than a destination. This model includes several key domains: (a) promoting a culture and language of hope and optimism; (b) being "person-first" and holistic; (c) supporting personal recovery; (d) environmental support and commitment; and (e) action on social inclusion and the social determinants of health, mental health, and wellbeing (Jacob, 2015). Kidd et al. (2011) conducted a study on a recovery-based approach called Assertive Community Treatment, which involves a multidisciplinary team providing services for SMI clients in community settings. Using the Recovery Self-Assessment tool (O'Connell et al., 2005) to measure client outcomes (e.g., legal involvement, hospital days and episodes, housing, employment, and education), researchers gathered data from multiple Assertive Community Treatment teams in Ontario, Canada ($n = 79$) that included data from 1,400 SMI client participants who received this treatment. Using multiple regression to analyze data, Kidd et al. (2011) found significant relationships between receiving treatment and less legal involvement ($r = .37, p < .01$), less hospital days ($r = .28, p < .05$), and more participation in formal education ($r = .28, p < .05$). Although the other outcomes did not have significant correlations with treatment, the overall model was significant, indicating that this treatment had an impact for clients ($F = 2.86, R_2 = .14, p < .05$). Although the sample was both limited and too broad (i.e., the sample was restricted to one geographic location, and included SMI clients ranging in diagnoses), this study provided evidence that the recovery model has the potential to produce meaningful outcomes for clients.

Overall, the evidence for using positive psychology interventions with people with psychosis is promising. Although there are multiple specific interventions that have been used by clinicians and reviewed in the literature described here, these treatments share overarching themes of focusing on clients' strengths, resilience, and often helping them foster positive relationships and develop meaningful self-narratives. Outcomes across studies include increased resilience and self-esteem as well as decreased symptoms and distress. With this evidence in mind, therapists may consider

implementing strengths-based approaches in their work with people with psychosis and

people who hear voices. Next, I shift to a review of the current literature on clinicians'

perspectives of people with psychotic experiences to highlight what is presently

understood and believed about this population among mental health professionals.

Therapist Perspectives of People with Psychosis

In recent years, there has been an increase in interest on research in how people

with psychosis view the cause of their psychotic experiences, but little is presently known

about what clinicians believe about these experiences (Carter et al., 2017; Saayman,

2017).

Ahn et al. (2009) found that providers perceive different mental health problems

as the result of different factors, with schizophrenia being classified as the most

"biological" of all disorders. This study used a sample ($N = 89$) of participants with

occupations including psychiatrists ($n = 20$), psychologists ($n = 20$), clinical social

workers ($n = 19$), psychiatry residents ($n = 10$), psychology interns and clinical graduate

students ($n = 10$), and social work fellows ($n = 10$). The participants completed

questionnaires designed by the researchers to rate their familiarity with all mental

disorders in the DSM-IV-TR (APA, 2000), as well as to rate the extent to which they

believe the disorders are biologically, psychologically, or environmentally based.

The majority of clinicians in this study conceptualized mental health problems as

predominantly psychosocial *or* environmental, failing to use an integrated approach.

Additionally, practitioners received different training specific to their professional group.

This training may have kept them focused in their area of expertise and not provided a comprehensive representation about beliefs about etiology across disciplines. Ahn and colleagues' (2009) study demonstrated that differences in etiological beliefs exist among different service providers; however, it did not provide specific information about the different types of training within each specialty. For example, the licensed psychologists as well as psychology interns and clinical students were not identified in terms of their training coming from a clinical, counseling, or other psychology program. A study that looks at these experiences could provide more informative data about how training impacts clinician beliefs and experiences in practice.

A study by Carter and colleagues (2017) examined clinician beliefs about the causes of psychosis. They noted how the integrated approach has been largely accepted in recent years, leading to clinical guidelines (NICE, 2014) advocating for a combination of antipsychotic medication and psychosocial interventions. Carter et al. measured practitioners' beliefs about the etiology of psychosis, the treatment offered to clients, and opinions about the helpfulness of these treatments. This study took place in the United Kingdom and surveyed a sample of 219 practitioners across a range of helping professions (CPN; social worker; psychiatrist; staff nurse; care coordinator; psychologist; team manager; occupational therapist; support workers; and other).

Carter et al. (2017) found that clinicians across the sample reported offering both psychological and pharmacological treatments but were more than twice as likely to offer medication compared to CBT (85% prescribed antipsychotic medication, whereas 40% were offered CBT). This study also found results that contradicted those found by Ahn et al. (2009) in which clinicians adopted a multi-causal, integrative approach in conceptualizing their clients. Also deviating from prior studies, Carter et al. (2017) found that psychosocial factors were endorsed more frequently than genetic or biological

causes. The researchers predicted this may be because of recent developments and

advances in therapeutic techniques, and also because multiple studies in the past sampled

medically trained staff as opposed to a broad sample of practitioners. Another finding

was that participants' beliefs about psychosis tended to influence their endorsement of

different treatments. A belief that antipsychotic medication was helpful was positively

associated with endorsing the biomedical model of psychosis ($r = .413$, $p < 0.01$) and

negatively associated with endorsement of the psychosocial model of psychosis ($r = -$

$.153$, $p < 0.01$). A belief in the helpfulness of CBT was positively associated with

endorsing the psychosocial scale ($r = .244$, $p = 0.01$). Carter et al. (2017) concluded that

clinicians' etiological beliefs are likely shaped by the training process that is specific to

their profession. They also concluded that clinicians' etiological beliefs about psychosis

were associated with their perceptions about the helpfulness of treatment. If practitioners

endorsed psychosocial factors as being the primary cause of psychosis, they were likelier

to believe that CBT would be helpful, whereas those who endorsed the biomedical model

believed medication was more helpful. One important implication from this study was

that such a strong focus on the perceived cause may blind clinicians to the benefits of

additional or alternative treatments, as well as the effectiveness of positive psychology

interventions.

Although there is sparse literature on clinicians' beliefs about and experiences of

working with people with psychosis, Larsson et al. (2012) completed a qualitative study

that used a discourse analysis method to explore how counseling psychologists

experienced work with people with psychosis, and constructed diagnoses for psychotic disorders. The researchers interviewed eight counseling psychologists in the United

Kingdom using a semi-structured interview designed by the researchers. The authors

found that the counseling psychologists interviewed tended to construct their experiences

of working with people with psychosis in a relational way, by both relating to the

individual's experience and normalizing the experience. However, pathologizing

language was still present when the participants described working with their people with

psychosis clients. Larsson et al. (2012) concluded that counseling psychologists were

placed in a difficult space between two epistemological positions: one that advocates the

use of diagnostic categories, and another that encourages the clinician to understand

clients on their own terms without labels. The researchers of this study did not provide

information about the semi-structured interview design and acknowledged this as a study

limitation.

Although this study (Larsson et al., 2012) did provide some insight into how

counseling psychologists viewed their experiences with people with psychosis, it was

limited to one sample of clinicians in the United Kingdom. This study creates curiosity as

to how practitioners with a counseling psychology background compare with those with a

clinical psychology background in terms of their beliefs and experiences with people with

psychosis. Additionally, it did not explore clinicians' etiological beliefs about how

symptoms characteristic of psychosis develops. There is an opportunity to expand the

research in these areas by addressing these questions using an empirical

phenomenological method that interviews practitioners from counseling and clinical

psychology training backgrounds.

Jones and colleagues (2019) also identified that there is a lack of research focusing on the perspectives of practitioners in their work with people with psychosis. Specifically, these researchers conducted interviews and focus groups with community mental health providers ($N = 34$). Focus group and interview questions centered on what practitioners considered optimal engagement with their clients (e.g., through questions such as "please describe your approach to working with clients with psychosis" and "what do you think it means to engage with clients and their experiences?"). Participants were also questioned about their beliefs on challenges and barriers to working with people with psychosis. Jones et al. (2019) identified themes across interviews and focus groups regarding engagement, the current state of mental health services, and perceived barriers. Engagement themes included the importance of the therapeutic relationship and engaging with the subjective meaning of psychosis. Practitioners discussed the importance of engaging with the meaning of psychotic experiences, including clients' perceived connections to life events and spiritual or personal beliefs. This finding appears to share similarities with the concept of helping clients make meaning of their experiences (Dilks et al., 2012; Roe & Davidson, 2005.) In terms of the current state of mental health services, a key finding was that staff felt underprepared for working with people with psychosis due to lack of psychotic disorder training in their education programs.

This finding is particularly relevant to the present proposed study, as it highlights the lack of training in working with psychosis and associated symptoms. However, Jones et al. (2019) invited more specific research to follow up on this finding, as specific details of participants' training were absent. The sample included three clinical psychology interns, one clinical psychologist, five bachelor-level mental health workers, and the remainder of participants with degrees in social work, counseling, or nursing. This sample appeared to be diverse, but in doing so, lacked specificity and may have been too broad by including participants with widely varying levels of education. Additionally, practitioners with a counseling psychology background appeared to be absent from this study. Including practitioners from this training background and comparing them with clinicians of a clinical psychology background could provide relevant information to the gaps in training programs regarding people with psychosis and people who experience auditory verbal hallucinations.

Summary

Through a review of the literature, I identified several themes that led to further exploration as I designed and conducted my study. Specifically, a key theme includes the traditional, medical model approach of pathologizing psychotic symptoms versus using the client's strengths to help them make meaning of their experiences. Much of the work I have reviewed so far describes stigma of severe mental illness that can be perpetuated by clinicians in their conceptualization and treatment of these individuals. People with severe mental health disorders, including psychosis, are less understood by both providers and the general population (Li et al., 2019), and have experiences that may classify them as a marginalized group. The phenomenon of healthy people experiencing auditory verbal hallucinations absent of other symptoms shows that clinicians may "think outside the box" of pathology and conceptualize these experiences in a different way. Current popular treatments for psychosis include CBT (e.g., Kennedy & Xyrichis, 2017; Menon et al., 2017; Penn et al., 2009; Shawyer et al., 2012; Zimmermann et al., 2005), mindfulness (e.g., Aust & Bradshaw, 2017; Chadwick et al., 2009; Langer et al., 2012; Lopez-Navarro et al., 2015), peer support (e.g., Castelstein et al., 2008; Chien et al., 2019; Cook et al., 2012; Mahlke et al., 2017), and pharmacologic interventions. Although the extant literature appears to show support for each of these approaches, none of them shows superior efficacy to the others. Positive psychology interventions are a viable option for working with people with psychosis and have also been shown to demonstrate efficacy with this population (e.g., Boiler et al., 2013; Drvaric et al., 2015; Meyer et al., 2012; Schrank et al., 2016). The literature on therapists' perspectives of working with this population is relatively sparse (Jones et al., 2019), and could benefit from a study that investigates therapists' experiences, biases, and beliefs about this work. A question that remains is: How can providers develop sensitivity and competency in working with these individuals? This question may specifically focus on clinicians' pre-existing beliefs about people with psychosis and what approaches they have used in both conceptualizing and working with clients who experience symptoms typical of psychosis, including the experience of hearing voices.

There is a need for research on therapists' experiences of working with people with psychosis, as well as those who hear voices, and their view of these clients in the context of a strengths-based perspective. Using a critical theory framework to guide this research conceptualizes people with psychosis as a marginalized population and explores through data analysis the ways in which clinicians view both barriers and strengths in their clients' lives. This study involved collecting qualitative data from psychologists and psychology trainees about their experiences in working with people who hear voices and how they select interventions and view the prognoses of their clients. Further, this study evaluates to what degree a positive psychology or strengths-based perspective is used to guide the therapists' conceptualization of and work with clients with auditory verbal hallucinations. By including practitioners from both counseling and clinical psychology disciplines, this research may highlight unique perspectives among training experiences of clinicians with people who hear voices and have implications for incorporating positive psychology into education.

CHAPTER III

METHOD

This purpose of this study was to investigate how mental health practitioners (specifically, psychologists and psychology trainees) conceptualize clients who report experiences of auditory hallucinations, with attention to any components of a strengths-based or positive psychology perspective. To accomplish this aim, I conducted qualitative research. Specifically, I employed an empirical phenomenological method. Empirical phenomenology is explained below in greater detail, as well as the philosophical presuppositions that underlie this study. These explanations are followed by a discussion of the methodological structure of this study, which includes participant selection, researcher biases and training, procedure and interview format, and data analysis strategy. I begin this chapter by identifying my research questions, followed by a discussion of the rationale for using qualitative research (and more specifically, empirical phenomenology) to address the research topic. An outline of the procedures for sampling and data analysis follows, including a discussion of the empirical phenomenology method used to analyze data, guided by a critical theory lens.

Research Questions

My primary research questions that were addressed by this study included: (a) What are the experiences of clinicians in working with people with psychosis, specifically, people who experience hearing voices? (b) How do clinicians approach treatment planning with clients who hear voices? (c) How do clinicians feel about working with people who hear voices? Specifically, how do they think their own views affect their work with these clients; how do they feel that their clients may be affected by biases of others? Are they familiar with critical theory? (d) Are clinicians familiar with healthy voice-hearers? What do they believe differentiates healthy voice-hearers from people with psychosis? (e) How do psychologists and psychology trainees believe that their doctoral program (both education and training) prepared them for working with people who hear voices? (f) To what degree do clinicians incorporate elements of positive psychology in their beliefs, experiences, and treatment planning of clients who experience hearing voices? (g) What do practitioners believe recovery looks like for people who hear voices?

Rationale for Qualitative Research

When considering the most appropriate methodology for my study, I considered many factors that are described in the following sections. The first question that came to mind focused on the broad but central theme of what I was hoping to learn from my participants and if this information was best gathered from quantitative or qualitative methods. Quantitative research typically uses objective measures (e.g., surveys with multiple-choice or Likert scale responses) to collect data in a systematic, uniform manner. A strength of quantitative data collection is the ability to quantify experiences into uniform language, analyze data using statistical analyses, and draw conclusions about statistical significance of the research questions that were investigated. However, this method is not the best avenue of inquiry for all research questions. A drawback of using the quantitative approach is that experiences are reduced to quantified variables, and there is no space for hearing participants describe their experiences in their own terms. Qualitative research, however, employs methods that allow for more rich data collection from participants who can share their experiences without the risk of simplifying their responses.

Qualitative research is a term that encompasses a broad range of methodologies and philosophical paradigms. Because qualitative research is so diverse in its methods, providing a unified definition of qualitative research is challenging (Creswell, 2013). Rather, this type of research may be viewed as not having a fixed definition, but it may be viewed as an approach to inquiry that is always evolving (Denzin & Lincoln, 2005). However, despite differences across the multiple methods of qualitative inquiry, there are common features that are shared among each of these methods. Qualitative researchers study the world in its natural setting; attempting to make sense of phenomena in terms of the meanings that people assign to them. Additionally, they share the common features of locating the observer within the world and aiming to in some way transform the world (Denzin & Lincoln, 2005).

Qualitative research was the most appropriate selection for the research topic of this study. Presently, there is a lack of literature on therapist perspectives of people with psychosis and people who hear voices However, the majority of research that does exist employs quantitative methods to explore patterns among practitioner beliefs (Ahn et al.,

2009; Carter et al., 2017). Although the findings from these studies provide information on what clinicians believe about how beliefs were shaped about clients who experience auditory verbal hallucinations, there is opportunity to expand this work by investigating how they conceptualize and plan treatment with these clients, including those who may and may not qualify for a psychotic disorder diagnosis. Jones and colleagues (2019) applied qualitative methods to investigating practitioner perspectives of people with psychosis but focused on service provision and barriers to treatment. Using a qualitative research design that extends this research by incorporating questions about training and influence of positive psychology provided an opportunity to gather data that provides a rich, thick, description of practitioner beliefs and experiences.

Although quantitative methods are ideal approaches to addressing some research questions, other questions require more robust data collection that helps the researcher understand the context of a phenomenon. My research questions identified for this study acknowledged the unique experiences of clinicians and in turn, the unique experiences of their clients. Attempting to quantify data across participant responses may require collecting closed-ended (e.g. "yes or no" or Likert scale) responses from participants, which risks minimizing their experiences and missing the rich contextual data that can be gathered through a qualitative approach. Although I was interested in learning from individual experiences, I was also curious about similarities underlying the experiences of clinicians who work with clients who hear voices. I was interested in learning directly from mental health practitioners about their beliefs and experiences in working with people with psychosis.

Multiple types of qualitative research involve collecting information directly from participants and making sense of these data. For example, the narrative approach invites participants to engage in storytelling to share their experiences. Although this approach can allow the participants to share their experiences more fully through storytelling, I was less interested in collecting unstructured narratives. Rather, I aimed to use a semi-structured interview to learn about the experiences of my participants as they relate to the topic of working with people who hear voices. Another example of a qualitative method that can involve direct participant interview is the case study method in which one participant is identified and interviewed. The case study approach may produce rich data about an individual's experiences; however, this approach is typically limited to a single person. I was interested in learning about the experiences of multiple participants who may differ in their training and clinical experiences. Most importantly, a researcher using a phenomenological method appreciates multiple perspectives and uses these numerous perceptions to understand the essence of an experience. In the case of my study, the experience broadly referred to practitioners' work with people with psychosis. Using a phenomenological qualitative approach enabled me to acquire this rich data. Phenomenology is discussed in more detail below, followed by a focused discussion on empirical phenomenology and how this method best suited my research questions.

Phenomenology

Phenomenology may be defined as the reduction of individual experiences of a phenomenon down to a description of the universal "essence" of that thing (Creswell, 2013). The phenomenological method may be traced back to Edmund Husserl, an early German philosopher. Husserl defined phenomenology as "the careful description of experiences in the manner in which they are experienced by the subject" and stated that it "proposes to study the whole of our life of consciousness (Husserl, 1936/1990, p. 46)." Moran (2013) provided a great deal of information on Husserl and his role in founding the phenomenological method in a book chapter from the text *Philosophy of Mind: The Key Thinkers.* Husserl's contribution to philosophy was explicated as Moran (2013) reminded the reader that Husserl did not attempt to explain *how* humans exist as conscious, cognitive beings; rather, he described *what* is involved in conscious experience. Intentionality is identified as a core concept of Husserl's beliefs about consciousness. Husserl believed that studying the intentional correlation between act and object may gain access to the essence of mental states; this is part of the phenomenological approach (Husserl, 1936/1970, p. 57).

Husserl was interested in the interlocking connections of "layers" of our intentional life – into a single, unified framework which provides a space for unity and identity of a single consciousness; as well as enables participation in the shared, universal, rational (our cognitive) life. Husserl, then, may be described as a holist, viewing intentional life as an interconnected whole. He aimed to uncover the basic forms of conscious life in terms of essential features, and necessary structural interconnections. Inner perception (our own perception of conscious sensations such as feelings and thoughts) and outer perception (perceiving objects outside ourselves) are both accessible through shifting – for example, moving from seeing the tree (outer) to seeing that our seeing of the tree involves temporally changing profiles (inner).

Moran (2013) further illustrated this concept with another example; that when watching a film, a viewer can shift from being absorbed in the plot to examining the camera shots and technical filming elements of the movie. It is this freedom of shifting our stance that allows us to use phenomenology. The transcendental nature of phenomenology "reveals the natural attitude, which is unaware of itself as an attitude, by adopting the transcendental attitude, an attitude which sees objectivity as produced by the achievements of cooperating subjects (Moran, 2013, p. 44)." Other aspects of Husserl's view on perception were provided, including the acknowledgement that an object may be only perceived from one side, which provides an incomplete picture. Husserl's emphasis on empathy was also expressed in Moran's (2013) overview. Empathy, Husserl believed, is a form of transcendence, or a "bridge to the other." It allows one to share the experiences of another; the self, Husserl (1936/1970) argued, is never experienced without the other. Self and other are interwoven, and the presence of others is a necessary condition to experience objectivity.

Another aspect of phenomenology that is applied by some researchers is document phenomenology, a way of understanding the subject of study (which may be the participant) as a source of information, or as a document (Trace, 2016). Participants as sources of information may be viewed as tangible, whereas the experience of processing information may be viewed as intangible. In this sense, subjects of phenomenological study can be considered material objects that also provide information that is more abstract and open to interpretation (Lund, 2009). Using a phenomenological method, researchers can understand a "document" (or, their participants) as sources of information that are situated in context of time, place, and consciousness of the world (essentially, how that person is experienced by others and how they exist in their environment). Through this process, attention is drawn to the contextual setting in which participants are situated; this understanding provides a more holistic view of participants and their experiences.

Empirical Phenomenology

The empirical phenomenology approach explores human behavior, psychological experiences, and situations as they are lived by the individual (Fischer & Wertz, 1979). This method is considered empirical through its use of the researcher providing specific guidelines for data analysis that may be replicated by future researchers. Through outlining specific guidelines for how the research was conducted, other researchers may be able to clearly see how they might replicate the study and arrive at similar findings (Fischer & Wertz, 1979). Proponents of this method appreciate that reality is comprised of multiple perspectives and is experienced differently by all individuals; yet unified in that researchers can arrive at consensus about its essential aspects (Yennari, 2011). Expectations and presuppositions are acknowledged as being not only present, but important in interpreting research results, and helpful in forming the frame of reference from which the phenomenon might be understood (Yennari, 2011). The researcher employs a reflexive procedure of acknowledging a priori assumptions, reflecting, and explicating implicit assumptions. In doing this, the researcher makes his or her approach as specific and explicit as possible, allowing for future researchers to understand how the researcher arrived at his or her findings, and to replicate the study to the best of their ability. Aspers (2004) provided a useful outline of the steps a researcher could take in designing an empirical phenomenological study. This outline includes seven steps: (a) define the research question; (b) conduct a preliminary study; (c) choose a theory and use it as a scheme of reference; (d) study first-order constructs (and bracket the theories); (e)

93

construct second-order constructs; (f) check for unintended effects; and (g) relate the evidence to the scientific literature and the empirical field of study. These steps are outlined in greater detail below.

The first step in Aspers' (2004) guide to designing an empirical phenomenological study is to define the research question. The question may emerge from personal interests of the researcher, but the theory that is used when forming this question should be guided by the researchers' engagement in the field. The second step involves conducting a preliminary study to determine if it is possible to address the research question. Here, the researcher may interact with others in the field to determine if the question may be answered, or he or she may review academic texts to gather relevant information on the topic of interest (Aspers, 2004). Presently, I have reviewed academic texts to find information relevant to my research topic and have outlined the existing literature throughout Chapter 2. Strategic research decisions are made and modified during this stage. I have been engaged in the process of modifying strategic decisions through working with my book chairperson to narrow and define the focus of my study.

Critical Theory Framework

The third step in Aspers' (2004) empirical phenomenological guidelines states that the researcher must select a theory to guide the research. The theory must fit the empirical evidence and research question, which gives focus to the study. A theory provides the researcher with a lens through which to view complex issues, focusing attention on different parts of the data and providing a framework for data analysis (Reeves et al., 2008). For this study, critical theory was used to guide the research.

Critical theory, in broad terms, is interested in empowering people to transcend constraints that are socially placed on them due to marginalized identities (Creswell, 2013). Conducting research through a critical theory lens allows for an understanding of contextual factors experienced by participants, to better understand how learning and experiences are shaped by society (Merriam, 2009). At the core of critical theory is the acknowledgment of power and oppression as being key issues in the lives and realities of marginalized groups. Qualitative research that is guided by and interpreted through this critical lens aims to empower the oppressed subjects of the study from societal constraints, and move towards transformative social action (May, 1997).

Although the participants interviewed in this study were mental health professionals, the ultimate subjects of data collection will be people who hear voices. As described in the previous chapter, these individuals experience marginalization in multiple ways due to stigma of psychosis and the prevailing medical model structure of mental health services. Using critical theory as a guiding paradigm for this study has enabled me to consider the ways that Western society and psychology's reliance on the medical model have, and continue to, shape the experiences of people who experience hearing voices when collecting and analyzing my interview data. As the primary researcher, I maintained a reflexive journal and attended to my own biases and social locations as I collected and analyzed data. Through acknowledging the positions of power that myself, as a researcher, and my participants, as therapists, have in relation to the clients they spoke about, I was mindful of the disconnect that existed between me, my participants, and the people they speak about. More information about this reflexive process is outlined in the Data Analysis section of this chapter.

The remaining steps of Aspers' (2004) guidelines to conducting an empirical phenomenological study deal with data analysis. These steps will be briefly described here, then discussed in detail as they are relevant to my study in the Data Analysis section of this chapter. The fourth step that Aspers (2004) outlined is studying first-order constructs and bracketing the theories. This can include the researcher finding ways to study the actors that lead to better understanding them. Empirical phenomenology holds that scientific explanation should be grounded in first-order construction of the actors, which consists of participants' own words and meanings (Aspers, 2004). The fifth step in Aspers' approach to empirical phenomenology, then, is relating these first-order constructs to the second-order constructions of the researcher. In this step, the researcher combines data gathered from participants with the selected theory. The sixth step outlined by Aspers (2004) in empirical phenomenological research is checking for unintended effects. This action consists of the researcher incorporating and making meaning of all the data presented by the participants, including that which seems inconsequential to the participant. Participants may share information that they personally consider to be uninteresting or irrelevant; but in fact, the researcher may consider this meaningful data. The final step in Aspers' (2004) outline of empirical phenomenology is to relate the evidence to the scientific literature and the empirical field of study.

An empirical phenomenological approach was an appropriate choice for this research topic. This method allowed for the appreciation of multiple perspectives, or realities experienced by the clinicians who were interviewed. Still, common features that are shared by all participants were identified and described as the essence of their experiences. Employing an empirical phenomenological approach provides readers of

96

this study with a detailed outline of the procedures used, so that they may both understand how I arrived at my findings and may replicate the study to the best of their ability in the future.

Procedure

Sampling and Recruitment of Participants

Participants for this study were recruited through purposive sampling at community mental health agencies, college and university counseling centers, and hospital settings. They must have had experience working with at least one client who experienced auditory verbal hallucinations. It was not a requirement that these clients had a psychotic disorder diagnosis to allow for professionals who had experience working with healthy voice-hearers. Participants must have been licensed clinical or counseling psychologists, or postdoctoral fellows or predoctoral interns from clinical or counseling psychology programs. Participants were recruited by first reaching out to regional community mental health agencies and university counseling centers with an introductory e-mail (see Appendix B) introducing myself and the research project to the director of each agency. I selected these sites using my professional local network to identify locations that are within the northeast Ohio area. Agency directors forwarded the e-mail solicitation to clinicians or provided me with their direct contact information. Two participants were recruited using this method. As an adequate sample size was not obtained through this process, I utilized my professional networks and those of my book committee members to identify potential participants. Through this method, I gained one additional participant. Finally, I distributed my information by contacting members of APA Divisions 12 and 17 listservs. One member of Division 12 was also in a leadership role in Division 18, Psychologists in

Public Service. She shared my information with the Division 18 listserv. The remaining eleven participants were recruited through this method and completed the screening survey to indicate their interest.

Participants

Fourteen total participants took part in this study. The sample consisted of clinical psychologists ($n = 7$), counseling psychologists ($n = 2$), postdoctoral fellows from clinical psychology programs ($n = 2$), and predoctoral interns from counseling psychology programs ($n = 2$) and clinical psychology programs ($n = 1$). The sample consisted of participants who identified as female ($n = 9$) and male ($n = 5$). Participants were asked to describe their racial and ethnic identity in their own words when completing the initial participant survey. Participants described themselves as White or Caucasian ($n = 8$), Asian or Asian-American ($n = 2$), multiracial, mixed, or Latina/White ($n = 3$), and African American ($n = 1$). They worked in a diverse range of clinical settings, including psychiatric inpatient facilities, hospitals, or state hospitals ($n = 4$), VA medical centers ($n = 4$), private practice ($n = 3$), community mental health centers ($n = 2$), and a forensic outpatient setting ($n = 1$). The mean age of all participants was 44 years of age, and the ages ranged from 28 to 72, with 38 years as the median age. The table shown below provides the demographic data for each participant, including the pseudonym that was assigned to each for the purpose of this study.

Table 1

Participant Demographics

Pseudonym	Psychology Specialty	Position	Gender	Race	Current Setting	Age
Adam	Counseling	Psychologist	Male	White	Psychiatric inpatient facility	42
Deborah	Counseling	Psychologist	Female	White	Private practice	66
Marissa	Counseling	Intern	Female	Latina/White	VAMC	28
Amy	Counseling	Intern	Female	White	Hospital	28
Bruce	Clinical	Psychologist	Male	White	Private practice, forensic	71
William	Clinical	Psychologist	Male	White	Psychiatric inpatient facility	72
Sarah	Clinical	Psychologist	Female	Mixed	Community mental health center	53
Elizabeth	Clinical	Psychologist	Female	Asian	VAMC	33
Rachel	Clinical	Psychologist	Female	Asian-American	State hospital	40
Lisa	Clinical	Psychologist	Female	White	Private practice	35
Karen	Clinical	Psychologist	Female	White	Community mental health center, rural population	47
Jacob	Clinical	Postdoc	Male	White	Forensic setting	30
Alisha	Clinical	Postdoc	Female	African American	VAMC	35
Nicholas	Clinical	Intern	Male	Multiracial	VARC	30

Demographic Questionnaire. A screening questionnaire was administered to each potential participant prior to the interview through a survey website, SurveyMonkey (see Appendix C). This questionnaire gathered information about their specific discipline (e.g., counseling or clinical psychology), their licensure credentials, their education level, and the number of years they had been working as a therapist. Demographic information (e.g., gender, race, age) was also collected from individuals at this stage. Inclusion criteria were licensure in the mental health field as a psychologist, post-doctoral clinician, or doctoral level intern with training in clinical or counseling psychology, and past or present experience working with clients who experienced auditory verbal hallucinations. Participants who met these inclusion criteria and completed the survey were contacted using a follow-up e-mail from the primary researcher.

Individual Interview Protocol. The interview protocol for this study (see Appendix A) was developed using a semi-structured format to elicit open-ended responses from participants, while clearly addressing the identified research questions. This protocol was read aloud by the primary researcher in each interview. The protocol first asked participants about the typical populations they work with, then narrowed focus to asking about experiences with clients with psychosis or clients who hear voices. Each participant was asked to focus on a particular client with these experiences in detail, and to provide some demographic data on the client while maintaining confidentiality. The interview protocol then guided the researcher to ask participants if they were familiar with the concept of healthy-voice-hearers. If they were not, the researcher engaged in brief discussion about this topic. Participants were asked if they have experienced work with clients who fit this description, and what their beliefs were about these experiences. Participants were asked questions about stigma that clients who hear voices may experience, as well as asked to examine their own attitudes and biases towards this population. Finally, participants were asked to discuss familiarity with positive psychology, including to what degree they incorporated strengths-based approaches with clients who hear voices, and whether positive psychology was included in their educational training experiences.

Interviewing Participants

When the proposal for this study was first drafted, there were plans to allow participants to select between an in-person and a virtual interview through Zoom, a video conferencing website. Zoom is a platform with multiple security features to ensure the privacy of calls and shared content and has multiple security and privacy certifications (e.g., SOC2, TRUSTe, EU-US Privacy Shield, FedRAMP; Zoom, 2019). Due to social distancing restrictions per COVID-19 protocol, in-person interviews were not presented as an option, and Zoom was the primary medium for interviewing participants. Participants were provided with a small monetary incentive ($25 each) in exchange for their participatory time and effort. The interviews followed a semi-structured format and were designed by the primary researcher with feedback from the Chair and Methodologist. The projected number of participants interviewed were between 12-15 people; or until saturation was reached, and new information was no longer being collected (Glaser & Strauss, 1967). The final sample of participants consisted of fourteen clinicians. Each interview lasted around 45-50 minutes and was recorded with permission from the participants. A technological error occurred during an interview with the final participant,

Amy, and unfortunately her interview was not recorded. Her responses that are shared in this paper were transcribed from notes that I took during our interview.

Institutional Review Board (IRB) Approval

Approval to conduct this study was obtained from the Cleveland State University Institutional Review Board (IRB) prior to recruiting participants. Informed consent forms, the recruitment survey, and interview protocols were submitted to the IRB for review to ensure they were aligned with ethical standards for participant treatment. Prior to beginning the interviews, participants were additionally informed that their participation was voluntary and they could withdraw from the study at any time with no consequence. Each participant was assigned a pseudonym in order to protect confidentiality. The limits of confidentiality were discussed with the participants. This discussion included a disclaimer that although pseudonyms would be used for the name and employment location of participants, there was still a small risk that information they shared could reveal their identity to the audience of this study once the findings were published. Informing participants of this minimal but present risk allowed them to make informed decisions and share information honestly and willingly. To mitigate the potential risk, I used a form of member checking in which I clarified with each participant the information that they shared with me as I interpreted this information. Additionally, I engaged in member checking by verifying with each participant that they consented to my use of specific quotes.

Transcription of Interviews

Each interview was recorded using Zoom's recording mechanism. These recordings were confidential. Each interview was password-protected and saved to a secure, password-protected, encrypted laptop computer. Audio files were then transcribed by the researcher using orthographic transcription. Everything that was expressed by both the participant and interviewer was transcribed; including words, pauses, and utterances (Braun & Clarke, 2013). This method of transcription enriched the data by providing a detailed, accurate account of all parts of a participant's story.

Data Analysis

I maintained reflexive journals, field notes, and memos throughout both my observations and interviews, and referred back to them frequently during my interpretation of findings (Hays & Singh, 2013). This contributed to providing thick description of my study in that it developed an audit trail that I referred back to as evidence supporting my findings. I additionally engaged in a form of member checking in which I clarified participant responses, using probes when necessary throughout the interviews (Hays & Singh, 2013). As an additional method of checking my work, my methodologist checked my data coding.

Using Aspers' (2004) guidelines to empirical phenomenology, I used the steps that were outlined as part of data analysis: (a) studying first-order constructs and bracketing the theories; (b) constructing second-order constructs; (c) checking for unintended effects; and finally, (d) relating the evidence I found in my study to the existing scientific literature and situating my findings within the empirical field of study. For Aspers' (2004) data analysis step that involves studying first-order constructs and bracketing theories, I first considered "raw data," participants' interview responses and behaviors independent of any of my pre-existing knowledge, or biases drawn from theory. In the next of Aspers' (2004) data analysis steps, I constructed second-order constructs. This process involved developing constructs in relation to participants' first-

103

order constructs. These interpretations served as ways of making sense of the data and tying interview responses to existing theory while still honoring participants' understanding of a phenomenon. Next, I engaged in the sixth step of Aspers' (2004) empirical phenomenology guidelines and checked for unintended consequences. These consequences may have included parts of participants' stories that they may have found to be uninteresting or irrelevant, but that the researcher may have found to be connected to outcomes. Finally, the last step of Aspers' (2004) guidelines to conducting empirical phenomenological research is to relate the evidence to the scientific literature and the field of study. As I analyzed my data and began to form conclusions related to my topic, I viewed my results within the context of the extant literature in the field, as well as discussed ways in which my study will add to and enrich the available body of research.

Primary Researcher

I have an interest in working with people with psychosis, as well as understanding the experiences of these individuals. I am interested in learning from other mental health practitioners about their experiences working with both people with psychosis and healthy voice-hearers. I have worked in several community mental health agencies for six years through my practicum and internship experiences during both my master's and doctoral work. My educational and training background consists of a combination of clinical and counseling psychology, from my master's and doctoral level programs, respectively. This training has shaped my interest in highlighting some of the unique experiences in training programs and exploring how clinicians with different training backgrounds conceptualize and work with people with psychosis. Through reviewing the available literature on psychosis, I was intrigued by learning about the existence of healthy-voice-hearers, and the prevalence of auditory verbal hallucinations in people who do not otherwise meet criteria for a psychotic disorder diagnosis. Reading about experiences of otherwise healthy individuals who hear voices also strengthened my interest in working with people with psychosis and made me begin to question what can be learned about living with verbal hallucinations from clinicians who work with these clients.

My personal social locations may inform some of the ways that I view people with psychosis, as well as my work with clients in general. I am a White, heterosexual, cis-gender woman who has a college education including graduate training. I have had the opportunity to work with a variety of diverse clients throughout my emerging career. I continue to be aware of the privilege associated with these multiple identities, and how this provides me and my clients with different experiences of the world. I have had multiple opportunities in terms of employment and education that result in financial stability, which many of my clients have not experienced. Another piece of my identity that provides me with privilege compared to my clients is my lack of symptoms characteristic of a psychiatric disorder. Although I experienced adjustment disorder during early adolescence, I have never personally been to therapy in the role of the client and have not experienced my own difficulties with mental health in many years. Bearing this in mind, I realize that clients may perceive me as unfamiliar with their experiences, making it more difficult to build therapeutic rapport. This may be especially true of people with psychosis. Given the stigma that is associated with psychotic experiences, I believe that these individuals may be more reluctant to open up to a mental health provider who is personally unfamiliar with their symptoms.

Additionally, through my experiences at community agencies, I have had several opportunities to work with individuals who experience symptoms characteristic of a psychotic disorder, usually in the form of auditory verbal hallucinations. Through my most recent experience in a community mental health setting for children and adolescents, I have had the experience of conducting psychological assessment with young clients. Two testing cases that I previously worked on involved children who reported hearing auditory verbal hallucinations, each absent of all other symptoms that would qualify the individual for a psychotic disorder diagnosis. In each of these particular cases, testing revealed that the voices they experience stem not from psychosis, but from anxiety. The recommendations I provided to the therapists working with each of these clients shifted the focus from perceived deficits to a strengths-based perspective; highlighting strengths that I identified for each client and encouraging the clinicians to work with these strengths to build resilience and facilitate well-being. Conceptualizing these clients as people not experiencing schizophrenia or another psychotic disorder has expanded my awareness of what auditory verbal hallucinations may represent and mean for different individuals. I used this motivation for increased awareness and understanding of these experiences in my phenomenological work.

Summary

For this study, I used an hearing voices in terms of beliefs about psychosis and treatment planning for people with psychosis. A sample of both counseling and clinical psychologists and psychology trainees was recruited and interviewed about their beliefs, biases, and experiences. I gathered information about to what degree practitioners from both clinical and counseling backgrounds use strengths-based or positive psychology approaches with this population. This empirical phenomenological study used a critical theory lens to better understand the experiences of practitioners and the experiences of their clients within the context of a Western society that often perpetuates stigma for people with psychosis, and more specifically, people who experience hearing voices. This study can add to the literature on how people with psychosis are understood and treated by mental health workers of different training backgrounds and provide a fresh perspective on how both people who hear voices and their clinicians can experience more empowerment and understanding in a clinical setting.

CHAPTER IV

RESULTS

This qualitative phenomenological study involved collecting and analyzing clinicians' interview responses to answer the primary research questions. The central question guiding this study was: How do mental health practitioners conceptualize and plan work with clients who hear voices? Specific research questions included: (a) What are the experiences of clinicians in working with people with psychosis, specifically, people who experience hearing voices? (b) How do clinicians approach treatment planning with clients who hear voices? (c) How do clinicians feel about working with people who hear voices? Specifically, how do they think their own views affect their work with these clients; how do they feel that their clients may be affected by biases of others? Are they familiar with critical theory? (d) Are clinicians familiar with healthy voice-hearers? What do they believe differentiates healthy voice-hearers from people with psychosis? (e) How do psychologists and psychology trainees believe that their doctoral program (both education and training) prepared them for working with people who hear voices? (f) To what degree do clinicians incorporate elements of positive psychology in their beliefs, experiences, and treatment planning of clients who

108

experience hearing voices? (g) What do practitioners believe recovery looks like for people who hear voices?

The current chapter reviews the data and the identified themes that emerged within the data through the process of Aspers' (2004) guidelines to conducting empirical phenomenological research. The results are presented in the order of the interview questions that participants were asked. First-order constructs, which use raw data in the form of direct quotes from participants, are included for each question. Second-order constructs, which are comprised of my interpretations of the raw data, are included for each interview question as well. The themes that emerged from each section of the interviews are described throughout this chapter. Any unintended consequences (parts of participants' responses that I may find relevant to outcomes despite participants considering them irrelevant) are mentioned throughout the results section as well. Aspers' final step of data analysis, relating the results to the existing literature, will be reviewed in the discussion section (Chapter V) of this paper. In the current and following chapter, the terms "participants," "respondents," "clinicians," "practitioners," and "therapists," and "psychologists and psychology trainees" are used interchangeably to refer to the people who were interviewed for this project. The interview question topic, the emergent themes, and a brief narrative description of each are listed below in a table format as well.

Table 2

Interview Questions and Themes

Interview Question Topic	Themes	Narrative Description
Therapeutic Approach to working with People with Psychosis	Therapeutic Alliance	The therapeutic alliance was acknowledged as integral to therapy regardless of primary treatment approach
	Navigating the Context of the Medical Model	Many practitioners described their experiences of navigating clinical work in the context of the medical model
Clinicians' Feelings about Working with People who Hear Voices	Normalized View of Hearing Voices	Clinician opinions included a normalized, rather than pathologized, view of hearing voices
	Some Level of Challenge	Many clinicians admitted to experiencing some level of challenge in work with people who hear voices
	Clinician Biases	Clinicians did not discuss present biases, but many revealed former biases and acknowledged biases of others
Familiarity with Critical Theory	Familiarity with Related Concepts	Although most clinicians were unfamiliar with the term, many were familiar with related concepts
Healthy Voice-Hearers	Familiarity with the Concept, but not the Term	No participants were familiar with the term "healthy-voice hearers," but many were familiar with the concept

Interview Question Topic	Themes	Narrative Description
	Considering Voices in a Cultural Context	Many practitioners spoke about cultural factors they have taken into consideration with clients who hear voices
	Hearing Voices Network	Several participants described familiarity with the Hearing Voices Network, a global peer support community for people who hear voices
Clinical and Counseling Psychology Training	Clinical Psychology has Some, but Limited, Emphasis on Psychosis	Clinical psychology practitioners received some exposure to psychosis work in their doctoral programs, but less than expected
	Practical Experience Provided more Training than Coursework	Clinicians, regardless of education background, reported more experience with psychosis through clinical work than academic work
	Clinical Experience with Psychosis was Often a Choice	Students who were interested in working with people with psychosis were largely responsible for seeking out these opportunities
	Participants' Preparation for Psychosis Work	Clinicians felt that their doctoral programs had provided them with some, but not always adequate, preparation for working with psychosis
	Counseling Psychology Takes a Holistic Approach to Psychosis Work	Participants trained in counseling psychology reported taking a holistic approach to clinical work

Interview Question Topic	Themes	Narrative Description
Training and Familiarity with Positive Psychology	Counseling Psychology Emphasizes Positive Psychology	Counseling psychology clinicians endorsed familiarity with positive psychology
Implementing Positive Psychology in Their Work	Positive Psychology across Different Therapeutic Modalities	Several participants described emphasizing a client's strengths in treatment, regardless of their primary therapeutic approach
	Meaning-Making Involves Meeting Clients where They Are	Many participants believed meaning-making in therapy involves meeting the client where they are
Belief in Recovery	"Recovery" is Individualized and Often Non-Linear	Clinicians agreed that recovery is different for each client and often non-linear
	Recovery is Possible but May Not Involve Eliminating Voices	Participants agreed recovery is possible but does not necessarily involve a complete elimination of voices
	Recovery Involves Self-Advocacy and Social Supports	Many clinicians identified clients' abilities to advocate for themselves and social support as essential factors for successful recovery

Populations Served by Clinicians

The sample for this study involved fourteen total participants, including four clinicians from counseling psychology background and ten clinicians from clinical psychology backgrounds. Participants interviewed worked across a variety of clinical settings in their past and present. In terms of current work setting, clinicians reported working in hospital settings, including Veteran's Affairs Medical Centers (VAMC) and Veteran's Affairs Recovery Centers (VARC), state psychiatric hospitals, and the psychiatric unit at a general hospital. Several clinicians reported working presently in forensic settings, including the aforementioned state psychiatric hospitals, community mental health centers that serve forensic populations, and a private practice that provides forensic services. Community mental health centers as well as private practice settings were also reported as current sites where participants work. Clinicians' past work settings were also varied; residential treatment centers for children and adolescents, VAMCs, state forensic hospitals, psychiatric inpatient units in hospitals, community mental health centers, and college counseling centers were all listed as participants disclosed past clinical work settings. A table displayed below (Table 1) lists participants' current work settings along with demographic information, including gender, race/ethnicity, and age.

Participants' Case Study Vignettes. Each participant was asked to share a brief case study about a client they worked with who experienced hearing voices. This section of the results provides information about the participants' brief descriptions of their clients. Additional details about participants' perceptions of and approaches to working with these clients is reserved for a later section of this chapter.

Adam, a 42-year-old White male counseling psychologist who was working in a psychiatric inpatient facility, shared that he worked with a client who was a White male in his mid-thirties. This client heard critical voices that made negative statements such as, "You're a freak, nobody likes you." He was inclined to isolate himself socially and had intermittent suicidal ideation.

Deborah, a 66-year-old White female counseling psychologist working in private practice, shared a vignette of a female client whom she has been working with for about six years. This client first presented with post-traumatic stress symptoms, and after some time working with Deborah, became paranoid about therapist notes and medical records. The client identified herself as being fragmented into parts and noted that some of her parts audibly spoke to her.

Marissa, a 28-year-old White and Latina female counseling psychology predoctoral intern who was completing her internship at a VAMC, reported on her work with a male client in his 50s who was diagnosed with schizoaffective disorder. He heard voices that he referred to as spirits, and he believed the spirits to be real and rejected his diagnostic label.

Amy, a White 28-year-old female counseling psychology predoctoral intern who was working in a hospital setting, described an experience with a cisgender, heterosexual Indian American woman in her 20s. This client was placed in the ICU for psychosis in the context of methamphetamine use, was distracted, paranoid, and internally stimulated, and had difficulty with abstraction.

Bruce, a 71-year-old White male clinical psychologist, worked in private practice with forensic clients. He reported on his work in a prior clinical setting with an adolescent boy who heard voices and experienced delusions about being audiotaped through the electrical sockets during therapy sessions.

William, a clinical psychologist who was White, male, and 72 years of age, most recently worked in a psychiatric inpatient facility. He described his work with a client who was in her mid-to-late-twenties, Caucasian, and female. She was repeatedly admitted to the hospital, discharged once stabilized, and then re-admitted. She heard voices that told her to harm or kill herself.

Sarah, age 53, described herself as a racially mixed female clinical psychologist who worked in a community mental health center. She described two client vignettes. One case involved a Black woman in her late 30s with whom Sarah worked in a pain clinic who heard a running commentary in her head describing what she was doing. Sarah's other case study involved a White female client in her 60s who used a wheelchair and was disabled. She believed she was a twelve-year-old boy and insisted that people refer to her as such. She also described this client as having an "OCD quality", as she was preoccupied with the details of her identity as the boy.

Elizabeth was as a 33-year-old Asian female psychologist with two licenses; she is licensed and works as both a clinical and a school psychologist. For the purposes of this interview, she selected her responses to focus on her clinical work at a VAMC setting. Her case vignette focused on a female client in her early forties who presented with a long history of the inability to maintain employment due to interpersonal difficulties. This client heard voices that were critical in nature, and the client was paranoid about her surroundings and other people as well, thinking that the juice was being poisoned and insisting that her juice boxes were served unopened to verify their safety.

Rachel, a female clinical psychologist who identified as Asian American and was 40 years of age, was working in a state hospital. She focused her brief case study on a client who was arrested for a violent crime. This client believed that voices took over his body, and that the voices were from people he had been in a gang with. He experienced the voices of these former gang members as being angry, mocking him, and threatening to kill him.

Lisa was a 35-year-old White clinical psychologist who was working in private practice. She described working with a 19-year-old client who was diagnosed with bipolar depression. Lisa described this client as having auditory, visual, and tactile hallucinations as features of their bipolar depression. Regarding the auditory hallucinations, this client would frequently hear scratching, growling, and banging noises that Lisa described as "scary and ominous."

Karen, a 47-year-old White female clinical psychologist, worked in a community mental health center serving a frontier population. She presented several client vignettes throughout the interview. One of these clients was a woman in her mid-sixties with whom Karen had been working on and off for eight years. This client had experienced abuse throughout her lifetime and began experiencing psychosis during her teenage years. Another client she described interpreted the voice she heard as being from God and found the voice to be a source of comfort. She also described another client, a woman who heard voices and interpreted them as angels. These voices originally spoke to her with faith-based affirmations, but eventually turned demonic. One of the voices told her that her cats were seriously ill, and the woman responded by drowning her cats in her bathtub, genuinely believing that she was helping them avoid a slower and more painful death.

Jacob was a 30-year-old White male postdoctoral fellow with a clinical psychology background. He was working in a forensic setting and shared a vignette of a client who was a 55-year-old man who looked older than his age. In response to his legal case, he was found to be not competent to stand trial and not restorable to competency, so was committed to the state hospital system and had been hospitalized for about twelve years.

He experienced delusions as well as heard voices (including the voice of his father) that regularly convinced him to stay at the hospital and warned him not to leave.

Alisha was a 35-year-old African American female postdoctoral fellow from a clinical psychology program who was working at a VAMC. The brief case study she shared was about a client with whom she worked when she was a case manager. This client heard command hallucinations and would present to sessions wearing earphones to block out the voices.

Finally, Nicholas was a 30-year-old multiracial predoctoral intern from a clinical psychology program and was working at a VARC. He shared an experience when he worked with a client he described as experiencing "meth-induced psychosis, where he would hear voices outside his body." This client believed the voices may be coming from the vents or standing behind him, "which resulted in some delusional thinking that it was coming from the government because they have the technology to do so."

Therapeutic Approach to Working with People with Psychosis

When asked to describe their approaches to working with people with psychosis, participants responded with varied modalities. Many respondents reported using therapeutic techniques from more than one theoretical framework, and none reported exclusively working from a manual in their interventions. Overwhelmingly, participants described their approaches as respecting the client and allowing clients some level of autonomy in their treatment. In terms of specific treatment approaches that were identified, answers included: CBT, ACT, DBT, psychodynamic, person-centered therapy, recovery-oriented therapy, and illness management and recovery. Although respondents expressed different primary approaches to treatment, shared components of their therapeutic approaches emerged from their interviews and are described below as common themes, including recognizing the importance of the therapeutic alliance and describing how they navigate the context of the medical model.

Therapeutic Alliance

The therapeutic alliance was acknowledged as integral to therapy by multiple clinicians regardless of their primary therapeutic approach. Part of the therapeutic alliance described by some participants involved the process of "joining with" the client, meeting them where they were, and normalizing, rather than pathologizing, their experiences. Bruce recalled an experience with a client he worked with in a forensic setting who believed that his "ocha," or power, had been stolen, and that he was committing crimes to regain a personal sense of power. At first, Bruce tried to utilize additional resources to help the client, and recalled:

> I had a priest that I came in contact with, who worked in a Spanish-speaking parish, and I tried to get the priest to hook me up with someone who could construct another power source for this guy. And I couldn't, we couldn't find somebody to do that.

Ultimately, Bruce worked on joining with this client, and described this approach to working with the client about his experience hearing voices:

> I essentially tried to join with him you know, I would talk to him, try to get him to, to detail, you know, how he was thinking about the voices, where they were coming from, um, who, you know, when did they begin?

Even if some clinicians did not describe "joining with" their clients, many of them described validation as a core component of their treatment approach. Two

118

participants who identified CBT as their primary approach reported using validation. Nicholas stated that depending on a client's level of insight, he may validate rather than challenge their experience. Rather than deciding if the client's experience is "real or fake," Nicholas and his client work together on how to manage distress from hearing voices. Rachel, another therapist who predominantly used CBT described taking a "curious approach to beliefs about their voices in addition to what the voices say," providing psychoeducation about hearing voices, and working to manage rather than fully eliminate the voices. She further described this curious approach as showing an interest in what clients believe about their voices, and said, "I want to explore the person's beliefs about their voices and their experiences with them and get to know the voices better." She also noted that CBT for psychosis involves normalizing experiences, and stated her belief that, "Under whatever circumstances, we all have the ability to hear voices at some point. We may have different thresholds." Jacob, who identified ACT as his primary treatment modality, emphasized the importance of building rapport regardless of a client's presenting problem. He described using grounding techniques to help the client focus on the present before "jumping into the delusions or the auditory hallucinations with them," and stated that rapport is needed before challenging psychosis. Alisha, a postdoctoral fellow with a clinical background described her approach as recovery oriented. She described that she tried to:

> ...kind of normalize it as much as possible to let them know like, okay, this is something that happens with a lot of people who have been diagnosed with this disorder. It's a disorder, doesn't mean that this is who you are. Your identity is not defined by this. You can still have an awesome quality of life. You know, you

hear voices and that just is what it is. So what are some ways that we can work through this or what has been working for you in the past? So it's really like having them define what are their goals, what they want.

Navigating the Context of the Medical Model

Evident across many interviews was an acknowledgement of the medical model and how clinicians navigate this model in the context of their work environments. These acknowledgements included participants' views of the medical model, and how they interact with medical providers to coordinate care. Adam, a counseling psychologist, described there being "two strands of psychiatry," where some clinicians only think about clients in terms of a medical approach, whereas others place a greater focus on psychotherapy. He then noted with disdain, "Hospitals are obviously for a lack of a better way of saying it run by physicians, right? Psychotherapy is an adjunct. It's not a primary treatment." When discussing her training in counseling psychology, Deborah noted how clinical psychology is moving towards using protocols, similar to medicine, "as if psychiatry was something like a pharmaceutical, which it's not." She noted how her paradigm changed over the years through working with clients and hearing similar themes emerge in their experiences. She stated that in her early career, she would have referred clients with psychosis to a psychiatrist, but no longer jumps to make that referral. Alternatively, Lisa, a clinical psychologist, reported that if a client presented with a primary diagnosis of a psychotic disorder, she would refer out to a specialist. Lisa stated that she only provided treatment to clients with psychosis if their psychotic symptoms were secondary features of their primary diagnosis, such as PTSD with psychotic features.

Multiple clinicians who were interviewed also identified their beliefs about the use of medication in clients with psychosis. All respondents who discussed the role of medication in treatment stated that they believed medication should not be the only ingredient in a client's treatment plan. Rather, some participants believed that medication was useful as an adjunct to, not a replacement for, psychotherapy. As Alicia, who described her approach as recovery-oriented noted, she encourages her clients to consult with the psychiatrist and be adherent with medication, but stated that she still honors client preference, and described herself as "still really being recovery-oriented and patient-centered." Other practitioners felt that medication is not always helpful and is not necessary for all people who experience psychotic symptoms. As Rachel noted, many people take antipsychotic medication with the goal to eliminate their auditory hallucinations completely. Maintaining a focus on completely eliminating the voices can send the client an "unhelpful message about voices being bad," which may lead to internalized stigma.

Clinicians' Feelings about Working with People who Hear Voices

Participants were asked to discuss their feelings about working with clients who hear voices. Further, they were asked to examine biases held by themselves as well as mental health practitioners in general, and how those biases may affect clinical work. All the participants who were interviewed claimed that they had positive feelings towards clinical work with people who hear voices, although several described some level of challenge. Additionally, none claimed that they held personal biases towards these clients currently, but all seemed to be aware of and willing to discuss the biases of other clinicians. Some participants were able to describe personal biases they had early in their training before gaining more experience and confidence working with this population.

Normalized View of Hearing Voices

Many clinicians reported that their opinions about people who hear voices included a normalized view of hearing voices, considering auditory verbal hallucinations as they would any other symptom. Several participants described themselves as being familiar with the Hearing Voices movement, which will be further detailed later in this chapter under the research question titled "Familiarity with Healthy Voice Hearers." The basic premise of this movement is that hearing voices should be normalized rather than pathologized and referred to as "hearing voices" rather than "auditory verbal hallucinations." Consistent with this non-pathologizing view, Deborah said, "I don't say 'auditory verbal hallucinations,' I say, 'hearing voices.'" She then continued to describe her belief about how anyone may be susceptible to hearing voices given their life circumstances, and stated, "Everything on earth breaks or shatters if it's under enough pressure. Atoms, bones, computer screens, if there's enough pressure… and there's something about the human psyche or the human spirit that does this same thing." Rachel agreed with the potentiality of any person to hear voices given a combination of circumstances, vulnerabilities, and genetics, and said, "From a CBT view, under whatever circumstances, we all have the ability to hear voices at some point. We might have different thresholds."

Some Level of Challenge

Although the general tone of participant responses about working with people with psychosis was positive, there were also clinicians who admitted to experiencing some level of challenge in this clinical work. For some, the challenge was present in assessing treatment progress and acknowledging that sometimes, progress is slower than the clinician would prefer. As Jacob said, work with people with psychosis is "a little frustrating at times because you're not going anywhere very fast, but I enjoy it." In order to meet the challenge, he stated that he adjusts his expectations based on where the client is in their treatment. Marissa agreed that work with clients with psychosis can be challenging, but she too enjoys the challenge. She noted that every client has a "right to fail," but granting clients that autonomy can be frustrating, because "we care about our patients and want to see them do well, so sometimes it's hard to hold back if it's not in their best interest." Karen spoke about the complex nature of this work and called clinical work with this population "exhausting… stressful, yet rewarding."

Clinician Biases

Part of describing their feelings on working with clients with psychosis and clients who hear voices involved participants speaking about any of their own biases with this population. Regarding this question, no participants interviewed admitted current personal biases, but some mentioned biases that they held earlier in their career before working with this population. Karen recalled an early experience with a friend who went through a "psychotic break," and that she was afraid of him before she began graduate school, citing stigma from the media as a primary source of her fear.

Other participants reported awareness of and experience with practitioners who hold biases towards people with psychosis that can affect treatment. Adam stated acceptance of the populations that clinicians work with is a "necessary prerequisite" to engaging in treatment, and noted, "If you're biased against psychosis, you may think you can mask it, but you can't, and can give it away through nonverbals. Even sick people are gonna know that you're uncomfortable with them and then they're not going to be able to work with you." He then emphasized the negative impact of clinician bias with the statement, "If you don't believe you're going to have an impact on people, you won't, if you do, you can." Amy agreed that bias affects work with clients and noted that bias can present itself through countertransference. Alisha noted that many clinicians do not have training in recovery-oriented models and cultural sensitivity, and that clients may experience practitioners' bias more if clinicians are more directive and treat clients "like this peon and you're the all-knowing savior or something."

Although some participants described their work with clients with psychosis as being a deliberate choice, they also stated that the choice to work with these clients is not shared by all practitioners; as Nicholas said, "A lot of people shy away from that type of population." Jacob cited stereotypes about people with psychosis being violent as a main factor that contributes to some clinicians' fear of this population. He recalled that during his internship, there were several other interns who were "terrified" of psychotic clients during a psychiatric unit rotation at a hospital and stated that they were convinced these clients were dangerous. He noted "instead of acknowledging their own shortcomings, were saying 'Oh well, these people are like just dangerous and crazy', and very much stigmatizing them." He also pointed out that their perceptions of these clients must have altered how they interacted with them, and further noted that, "A lot of people don't understand what a psychotic disorder is. It's a product of your training." Jacob described his work in a hospital setting as well and noted that "Staff burnout with nursing staff is

124

huge with this population. Other staff members might have some opinions and attitudes that the patient doesn't want to get better and they just aren't trying at all."

Familiarity with Critical Theory

Overwhelmingly, clinicians who were interviewed were unfamiliar with the term "critical theory." After asking each participant about their familiarity with critical theory, the theory was briefly explained to them as a framework that highlights difficulties faced by marginalized populations and empowers people to transcend these societal constraints while acknowledging the influences of power and oppression. Although participants stated they were unfamiliar with this theory by name, participants reported that they had some level of awareness about the concepts involved in critical theory once it was explained, and others were familiar with closely related theories. Several of these therapists stated that when they had received their doctoral training, critical theory was not present in the literature. One clinician expressed an interest in learning more about the theory and expressed curiosity and a desire to learn more.

Familiarity with Related Concepts

When asked the open-ended question, "What is your familiarity with critical theory?" many respondents stated that they did not recognize the term, but that they were familiar with some of the general principles of the theory but called it by a different name. Several practicing psychologists noted that the research had changed since they had been in school. As Bruce said, "I might call it something else. Tell me what it means. I told you I might call it something different." Deborah responded to the question with, "It didn't exist when I was in graduate school," but noted that she was somewhat familiar with critical race theory. When asked about familiarity with critical theory, William said,

125

"Possibly, but not with that phrasing? I have to confess that I'm a little too far removed to be as knowledgeable about emerging literature as I used to be."

Other participants did not describe themselves as being far removed from their education but noted some level of familiarity with related concepts or elements of the theory using different language. When asked about her familiarity with critical theory, Elizabeth responded, "As it's called? I might be familiar with it in some other way." After receiving an explanation of critical theory, she spoke about stigma against SMI clients, particularly focusing on beliefs that some practitioners have that people with psychosis exhibit more violence than the general population. Adam remarked that he had loose familiarity "with some sociology stuff," and guessed that critical theory looks at systems of oppression and how they influence our understanding of the world. Rachel was unfamiliar with the term "critical theory," but wondered if the Hearing Voices movement was related, calling the movement "more of a social justice model, as opposed to a psychological, support treatment model that psychologists are trained in." Alisha believed that she may be somewhat familiar with critical theory, responding, "A little bit, is that like tied to or connected to liberation psychology, like critical consciousness?" After receiving an explanation of critical theory, Bruce inquired, "Is it akin to institutional racism or something like that?" Finally, Karen stated that she was "not familiar with that exact theory," but believed that power differentials are real and acknowledged the importance of recognizing structural forces when conceptualizing clients.

Healthy Voice-Hearers

Clinicians who were interviewed were asked to describe their familiarity with healthy voice-hearers. None of the participants indicated a familiarity with the term healthy voice-hearers as it is presented in recent literature (e.g., Baumeister et al., 2017; van Os et al., 2008), but many of them were aware of people who hear voices but do not otherwise meet criteria for a psychotic disorder. A common theme that was found among interviews was an understanding of cultural significance that some people attribute to their experience of hearing voices. Another commonality shared by multiple participants was experience working with the Hearing Voices Network.

Familiarity with the Concept, but not the Term

When participants were asked to describe any familiarity they have with the term healthy voice-hearers, all fourteen participants expressed unfamiliarity with the term. When the concept was described to them as "people who hear voices but do not report distress and do not meet any diagnostic criteria," clinicians indicated that they were familiar with people who hear voices but do not have a psychotic disorder as a primary diagnosis, as well as people who hear voices but do not experience them as distressing. Sarah reported working with people who are "well stabilized and their voices don't really bother them. They're functioning all right." But as she noted, since they are on medication, they definitionally meet diagnostic criteria for a disorder. Jacob noted that he worked with clients who hear voices as symptoms of non-psychotic disorders (e.g., bipolar depression, PTSD). Several other practitioners recalled that they had worked with clients who heard voices resulting from substance use, so psychosis was not the primary feature of their diagnosis. Finally, several therapists pointed out that it would be difficult to come across healthy voice-hearers in clinical work, as they would not be motivated to seek treatment if they are not experiencing distress. As Nicholas explained, "I think the biggest difference is just the ability to manage those experiences and be able to function independently."

Considering Voices in a Cultural Context

Once participants began engaging in a discussion on people who may be considered healthy voice-hearers, several of them began speaking about cultural factors that they have taken into consideration when working with or thinking about people who hear voices. William opened his response with, "I've always believed in and communicated … there are many communities or cultures or subcultures where hearing voices is normalized and supported and validated." He then provided an example from his personal life of a Latina friend's experience with hearing voices:

> I remember speaking with her awhile back and she said… in her family and in her community, it was considered a positive sign if you heard… deceased members of your family, talking to you and giving encouragement and guiding you. So she said, she remembers as a child, her mother telling her, you know, that her mother's grandparents visited her yesterday and they were talking and that she said I had an actual conversation and I felt that I was being responded to.

William then continued by describing that when his friend came to the United States and considered herself to be acculturated, she resisted some of these cultural beliefs about hearing voices that her mother continued to uphold. He continued with a quote from his friend,

'You know, mom in the US in [Redacted], we don't talk about talking to dead people or having people talk to us. Not that it's not believable, but you know, you have to adapt to the prevailing community and culture.' And she said, 'I was young enough when I grew up with my mother and my grandmother who passed away when she was an adolescent, that was not emphasized as much as it was when my mother was growing up so that I didn't have to unlearn in a sense, you know, the value and the honor of having members of your family who were gone, continue to communicate with you.'

Sarah also noted cultural differences that some clients may present with. She reported that she had experience working with Hispanic clients who were opposed to mental health interventions, but noted, "They usually, if they do hear anything, they do put it in a religious context and they tend to reject any diagnosis." Jacob also acknowledged clients' religious and cultural beliefs regarding voices and recalled a religious client he worked with who felt comforted by hearing the voice of God. He added, "I'm really careful about overpathologizing a spiritual or cultural experience." Bruce agreed with respecting cultural differences, and noted, "I know that there's some cultural kinds of experiences that people had or have that are more spiritually akin. Sometimes people hear the voices of dead relatives. I don't necessarily think that's a mental illness."

Hearing Voices Network

As participants described their experiences with healthy voice-hearers, four of the interviewed clinicians mentioned familiarity with the Hearing Voices Network. This network is a global peer community of people who hear voices, with different groups that have formed throughout the world. Although many of the groups are peer-led in a format similar to twelve-step programs, other groups involve facilitation by trusted mental health professionals. Their mission includes aiming to raise awareness of the diversity of experiences with voices, challenging stereotypes, and stigma, and encouraging a positive response to voice-hearing and related experiences in healthcare settings.

Two of the participants who mentioned the Hearing Voices Network reported that they had facilitated Hearing Voices groups in clinical settings. Amy reported that she facilitated a Hearing Voices group at a previous practicum site. Rachel, who also ran Hearing Voices groups Voices as,

> It's not a treatment, it's not a therapy, it's considered a human rights movement. And so they're not concerned with like whether or not Hearing Voices groups are empirically validated or effective. It's like, why do we need to prove that this is effective because it's not a treatment? Because it's a human rights issue and we're advocating for voice hearers and saying that this is, you know, that there's nothing wrong with voice hearing. So I think that, they fully, I mean, it's peer-led, it fully embraces that sort of more of a social rights, social justice model, as opposed to more, like a psychological, really supported treatment model that often psychologists are trained in.

Rachel described her view of hearing voices as a "variance of experience that a lot of us can eventually hear depending on stress, vulnerabilities, and genetics and all those things and how they interact." She shared a personal example of living with a healthy voice-hearer and said that her husband hears voices but is functional, employed, and does not currently experience significant distress. She described how his approach to managing the voices was to speak back to them in a compassionate manner, using his Buddhist studies as a guide:

> They were really mean voices and he started telling them, 'I, you know, accept you, I appreciate what you're doing.' And they would, you know, 'F you!' and get really angry, and he would just start talking to them in a more compassionate way that he kind of learned from just studying, you know, Buddhism. And they started to change and he just kept telling them I appreciate you. I love you. You're a part of me. And then eventually the voices stopped being so angry and they started being more helpful and they started saying things like, 'Don't forget to turn off the stove' and he would just thank them and they changed and eventually they went away.

Two other clinicians mentioned the Hearing Voices Network when asked about their familiarity with healthy voice-hearers, although they did not report experience with facilitating groups. Deborah noted that she uses the language of the movement and says, "hearing voices" rather than "auditory verbal hallucinations." She also suggested that hearing voices may be viewed on a continuum, "from exceptionally positive like 'You can do it!', you know, things that we've internalized as little kids … and that's sort of a voice it's not really auditory it's self-talk, but some self-talk could be viewed as somewhat auditory." She and Rachel also mentioned psychologist Eleanor Longden's TED Talk where she reveals how she views her personal experience with hearing voices as a positive rather than pathological attribute. Finally, Adam mentioned the Hearing Voices Network, and described it as an "organization that is more dedicated to making meaning out of voices." He also remarked that he believed this movement to be more accepted in Europe, and said, "I think it's kind of something they're more comfortable with in Europe, for example, and they do a lot more of it."

Clinical and Counseling Psychology Training

The sample of participants involved four clinicians from counseling psychology backgrounds and ten practitioners from clinical psychology backgrounds. Although both clinical and counseling psychology programs provide training for students to become licensed psychologists, programs are structured differently based on core principles of each specialty. Historically, counseling psychologists worked in vocational guidance roles and with clients with less severe mental illness than clinical psychologists (Delgado-Romero et al., 2012). Clinical psychologists have historically used the medical disease model to pathologize and "fix" clients' deficits (Yip, 2005). Presently, counseling psychology is defined as a specialty that "facilitates personal and interpersonal functioning across the lifespan with a focus on emotional, social, work related, educational, health-related, developmental, and organizational concerns (Council of Specialties in Professional Psychology, 2019)," and clinical psychology is defined as "a general practice and health service provider specialty" where clinicians "assess, diagnose, predict, prevent, and treat psychopathology, mental disorders, and other individual or group problems to improve behavior adjustment, adaptation, personal effectiveness and satisfaction (Council of Specialties in Professional Psychology, 2019)." Clinical psychology programs traditionally involve coursework on diagnostics, assessment, and psychopathology, and counseling psychology programs may emphasize coursework on lifespan development and career counseling.

In this section, information will be presented about participants' experiences in receiving doctoral coursework in working with clients with psychosis, as well as their beliefs about how their training in counseling or clinical psychology affects their work with people who hear voices. The emergent themes in response to this question included: clinical psychology programs provide some (but less than expected) training on psychosis; participants received more experience working with psychosis through practicum than coursework; getting experience working with psychosis was often elective; clinical psychology practitioners felt somewhat prepared to work with people with psychosis; and counseling psychology practitioners take a holistic approach to working with people with psychosis.

Clinical Psychology has Some, but Limited, Emphasis on Psychosis

When participants were asked to describe any training that they received through their doctoral program specific to psychotic symptoms or disorders, practitioners from clinical psychology programs generally reported that they received some coursework in this area, although this experience was not shared by all clinical practitioners. For example, Jacob reported taking a class that focused on SMI populations or psychopathology, and Sarah responded she took a one-credit class in "radical psychotherapy with schizophrenics," although noted she does not believe the course is presently offered. She remarked about the course,

> It was a total acceptance type therapy, you know, where you just like, just accept the delusion, go into the delusion and talk within the delusion, you know? And that was a long time ago. I don't know if it's offered anymore, if it's been debunked, but it was in the eighties, maybe nineties.

Four participants from clinical backgrounds reported that they had at least one class that focused on diagnostics and understanding the DSM. Two clinical psychology participants recalled taking an assessment course that included at least an overview of screening for psychosis. Two other clinical psychology-trained clinicians reported learning about psychosis through classes in a less direct way; one respondent took a class on evidence-based practice where she believes psychosis treatment was included; another clinician noted that they had "little to no coursework in SMI besides biological bases of behavior," and no classes that discussed treatment for clients with psychosis. One other therapist from a clinical psychology background remarked that they did not recall receiving any coursework that emphasized work with people with psychosis.

Participants with counseling psychology backgrounds reported that they did not receive much education on psychosis through their doctoral programs. Two of these participants recalled receiving "nothing" and about psychosis in their coursework. Two others reported "no formal training" and that their discussions about psychosis in school were "very limited," but acknowledged that these diagnoses and experiences were briefly reviewed in their diagnostic classes.

Practical Experience Provided more Training than Coursework

Regardless of clinical or counseling background, participants overwhelmingly indicated that they received more experience with psychosis in general through engaging in clinical work in their practicum placements. William noted that the training he received through his practicum experience was good, but the clinical psychology coursework was "all academic book learning. My coursework didn't really prepare me to work with psychotic clients that was, you know, in-vivo, seat-of-pants learning." Alisha pointed out that her Master's program provided more training in psychosis than did her clinical doctoral program, as the latter was more generalist than specialized. She also noted "the majority of my training was hands-on." Sarah agreed and emphasized that academia and practical experience are "almost like two separate worlds," but acknowledged the importance of the academic training, and stated, "you have to have the experience, but you need that background, you know, in theory." Overall, participants spoke about their clinical work as being more enriching and providing them with the opportunity to work with clients with psychosis compared to the education they received in their doctoral classes.

Clinical Experience with Psychosis was Often a Choice

Just as many clinicians reported that their practicum experiences were responsible for much of their training in working with people with psychosis, several of them also stated that students who were interested in working with this population were responsible for seeking out these experiences. Alisha, who noted that her doctoral program was generalist, stated that she intentionally chose practicum sites that emphasized work with clients with psychosis because that aligned with her interests. Elizabeth agreed that students were responsible for seeking out experiences with chosen populations, including clients with psychosis. She said, "They put the burden on the students to try and kind of navigate where they wanted to have their training in." Amy stated that the counseling psychology doctoral program she is currently enrolled in encourages students to "take our own paths of interest."

When asked about how they believed their doctoral training in either counseling or clinical psychology affects their work with people with psychosis, some participants reported feeling somewhat prepared for this work from their classes, but many stated that coursework alone did not adequately prepare them for clinical work. Bruce, a clinical psychologist, described that taking classes that focused on biology and psychopharmacology prepared him for working with this population. Rachel reported many of her clinical psychology classes emphasized the use of CBT, and that this approach prepared her to work with any population, including people with psychosis. She stated that most of her CBT work focused on helping clients with symptom management, and this focus was true for people with psychosis as well. Alisha, who was also from a clinical background, cited her coursework in abnormal psychology as being helpful to recall as she worked with SMI populations, although she noted (as detailed in a previous paragraph) that her classes did not provide as much exposure to psychosis as did her practicum experience. Similarly, Elizabeth had previously noted that she received limited coursework specific to psychosis, but still cited her training as being helpful in her work with this population. When asked about the influence from her clinical psychology training, she responded: "I think that's really important. It's really beneficial since it helps ground the framework and theory and conceptualize how I all believe about their cognitions, their behaviors and things like that." Although as noted in a prior section, even practitioners from clinical programs tended to report a lack of education specific to psychosis, the training that they did receive prepared them somewhat to work with people with psychosis.

Practitioners from counseling psychology training programs also reported that their coursework alone did not provide adequate preparation for work with these clients. As Marissa recalled, "I was a lot more reserved and kind of let clients have the majority of the session just because I didn't have that prior training experience." She further noted that training she received on building coping skills and healthy social supports generalized well, but she did not receive social skills training that is specific to clinical work with SMI clients. Deborah noted that she did not receive any education in her counseling psychology program specific to psychosis, so when encountering clients who experienced auditory verbal hallucinations or other psychosis symptoms, she was instructed to "refer to a psychiatrist." Similar to participants from clinical programs, those from counseling programs reported that they received most of their training in this area through practicum experiences.

Counseling Psychology Takes a Holistic Approach to Psychosis Work

Practitioners who were trained in counseling psychology conceptualized clients, including people with psychosis, using a holistic framework, and considered contextual factors and intersecting identities with their clients. Amy, a current predoctoral intern in a counseling psychology program, emphasized that the foundational principles of counseling psychology and how the "whole-person, intersectional, multicultural framework" is helpful for work with all her clients. She noted that professors in her program encouraged her to be holistic in case conceptualization, including considering all identities and symptom presentations. In her view, the broad lens and framework provided by her lessons in counseling psychology helped prepare her to "see a person as a person rather than reduce them to a diagnosis." Adam spoke about the attention to systems and the ways that biases can impact people that he learned through his program. When asked about how counseling psychology influenced his work with people with psychosis, he said,

> Certainly I think that in counseling psychology, you do have that attention to systems, right. And then, you know, the way that bias can impact people. I do pay attention to that when I'm dealing with people with psychotic disorders, which not everybody does.

Deborah contrasted clinical psychology's adherence to protocols and manualized treatments with counseling psychology's focus on understanding the client in the context of their environment and said: "I tend to speak to my clients rather than speaking to the academic literature."

In addition to counseling psychology clinicians' holistic view of clients, there was also some pride about their field of study that emerged in response to how their training influenced their work, particularly regarding the identity of being a counseling psychologist. Deborah said, "We're getting a little bit more assertive, more spunky, in defining ourselves." She continued by borrowing a quote, "We work with individuals through the lens of their lived experience rather than saying what we don't do," and added her own insight, "There's a need for that. Pick an environment, any environment, pick a marginalized population, any marginalized population, or for that matter, really wealthy people who are trafficked as kids… ranges over a quite wide range." William, a clinical psychologist, had some personal experience with receiving counseling psychology training, as one of his supervisors had this background and shared it with him. He described how his supervisor's viewpoints helped to shape his work with clients as well, and echoed the "spunky," assertive nature described by Deborah. He stated:

> One of my best supervisors came from a counseling psych program. And she said, 'Here's the difference between clinical psych and counseling psych. And here's what makes us better. Clinical psych only looks at what's not working, what the problems are, what needs to be changed. Counseling psych approaches the individual, what's working? What can we take from your day-to-day functioning and generalize it into areas where you're not having success? So don't start with the problems, start with the competencies.'

Training and Familiarity with Positive Psychology

During the interview, clinicians were asked an open-ended question about describing any familiarity they have with positive psychology. After disclosing what they know about positive psychology in general, participants were then asked more specific questions about how they may apply elements of positive psychology (e.g., a strengths-based approach, meaning-making) to their clinical work. If participants required further clarification, positive psychology interventions were described to them as emphasizing a client's strengths to solve problems or build resilience, or helping clients make meaning of their experiences. Results from these more specific prompts are detailed after the theme of familiarity with positive psychology based on doctoral program is described.

Counseling Psychology Emphasizes Positive Psychology

Clinical Psychology Training/Graduates. Clinicians who were interviewed were asked to describe their familiarity with positive psychology. Several clinicians who reported some familiarity with positive psychology recalled that they received some form of this training in their doctoral program, even if it was not emphasized. Lisa, a clinical psychologist, said,

> That was probably mentioned in our, um, just like general education, like clinical interactions or something … they like went through different types of therapy. So I'm sure... I mean, I know what it is, so I'm sure we did learn about, I don't remember what class or more specific about it.

Alisha agreed that she was familiar with positive psychology but noted that in order to learn about it in her program, students had to seek out that opportunity. She stated that she mostly gained familiarity through clinical work, and said, "I would say that is a huge component of the type of work that is done, like in the settings that I work in now and in practicum sites, like I didn't have formal coursework on that, but that was just like the style." Elizabeth reported that she did not receive education in this area but noted that a student in her clinical program selected positive psychology as a research area but had to take the initiative. Elizabeth was able to name Martin Seligman, a leader in positive psychology, but immediately followed with, "I know enough to know I don't know anything," and reported a lack of education on positive psychology. Additionally, Sarah, who is also from a clinical background denied that her program offered positive psychology education but stated that she had the opportunity to sit in on a lesson on positive psychology in her college counseling center practicum site.

Counseling Psychology Training/Graduates. Each of the participants who received training in counseling psychology doctoral programs reported at least some familiarity with positive psychology, and several indicated that they received some education specific to this area in their studies. Adam recalled learning about Martin

Seligman (2002) and understood positive psychology to be "a defining pillar of counseling psychology," but could not recall specific details of the approach. Amy described her familiarity with positive psychology as "fair, good" and reported that students in her program are encouraged to use a strengths-based approach with clients. Marissa endorsed "a bit" of familiarity with the approach. She noted that it was taught during her Master's program, but not in her doctorate program. Finally, Deborah reported being "very familiar" with positive psychology but noted that the term did not exist when she was in school, as she received doctoral training prior to the positive psychology movement. William, a clinical psychologist, echoed this experience, saying that he took classes prior to the movement, but noted that "positive psychology is something that I think has been emphasized with different labels throughout my training."

Implementing Positive Psychology in Their Work

Clinicians were asked to describe any elements of positive psychology that they may use in their work with clients who hear voices. They were also asked specifically to identify any cases where they emphasized a client's strengths in their work, as well as any elements of meaning-making they used in their therapeutic approach. All participants believed themselves to use at least some elements of positive psychology in their work, even if they did not initially identify these therapeutic techniques as being influenced by or related to positive psychology. Even for participants who had not identified familiarity with positive psychology (as discussed in the above section), each clinician was able to connect at least some piece of their clinical work with positive psychology, such as using client strengths and helping clients make meaning of their

141

experiences. Further, an emergent theme is that practitioners believed that helping clients make meaning of their experiences involves meeting them where they are.

Positive Psychology across Different Therapeutic Modalities

Several participants described emphasizing a client's strengths in treatment, even if the techniques they used stemmed from a different therapeutic approach than positive psychology. For example, Nicholas, Jacob, and Amy described using an ACT framework, and Lisa stated that she uses DBT with all clients. As Jacob mentioned, he uses an ACT framework and value-driven work and mentioned validating any strengths a client demonstrates in session, such as having the ability to identify emotions. He noted that he at first would not have associated positive psychology with his work, although he noted the similarities, and stated his approach was "a bit away from positive psych, but not entirely." Amy and Nicholas also noted that they use an ACT framework and incorporate values into their clinical work.

Two clinicians specifically used the term "recovery-oriented" as well as "person-centered" when describing how they use a client's strengths in treatment. Elizabeth described her approach as using "person-centered, supportive, recovery-oriented techniques," and that she uses "story narrative-centered" techniques with clients and encourages them to tell their own stories about their experiences. Alisha also described her approach as both person-centered and recovery-oriented. She described the importance of considering contextual factors for each client, including viewing social and family support as a strength for clients from cultures that value collectivist values. She described her role in highlighting these supports, "I point these things out as much as I can just to empower the person and not let them feel defined by the diagnosis, the symptoms, like give them hope."

Finally, other clinicians also endorsed a use of client strengths in their treatment with clients, including those who hear voices. Bruce spoke about being responsible for starting a mental health court and a drug court that provided strengths-based programs as a sentencing alternative. He described his experience,

> I worked in the criminal justice system for almost 30 years and what we get there because the mental health systems fail… we end up with people with mental illness that shouldn't be arrested and should be in hospitals or community mental health centers.

He described how the mental health and drug courts allowed for these clients to be diverted to a treatment program rather than spend time in a jail or prison setting. His strengths-based work with these courts was described as, "We did assessments on folks and tried to figure out what they were good at and try to enhance those kinds of characteristics as opposed to punishing and attempting to kind of remove more adverse aspects of their personality." Deborah described her approach as being "insight-oriented," and paused before she noted, "It could be framed as positive psych." Finally, Sarah reported that she had focused on clients' strengths before, and noted, "I do try to focus on what they bring to the table," which has included focusing on the fact that a client may be a survivor and demonstrate resilience.

Meaning-Making Involves Meeting Clients where They Are

Many of the clinicians who were interviewed responded to a question about helping clients make meaning of their experiences affirmatively and stated that they helped clients who hear voices make meaning of their experiences. A common theme that was identified across these respondents' answers was that using meaning-making in therapy involves meeting the client where they are. Jacob noted that he tries to help clients understand and express their values, and then work with them based on what is important to them. He said:

> I think that it really is saying, okay, what is it that you want? You know, like what is your goal? What are the things that matter to you? I certainly have used the value card sort and then say like, 'Okay, let's choose one of these. You said this is really important. How do you, what can we do to get you there?

He then continued by describing how this values assessment was used in treatment:

> …really linking it to kind of behavioral practical solutions in terms of what, whatever it is they want to do. So like with, you know, the guy who was experiencing auditory hallucinations, my work with him wasn't necessarily as value-driven because this is   somebody who wanted to stay in the hospital. So it was something more like, 'Okay, well you like going for walks. So what do you say if we go for walks?' And he was like, 'Okay, yeah, I do like going outside.' So we go for walks and that wasn't necessarily, you know, central to his values, but it was central to what the treatment team wanted, which is they wanted him to be more comfortable with the idea of leaving the unit with the idea of leaving the facility. So you know, we do a walk and we try to get closer to that road… every time didn't usually happen, but we certainly would try."

Marissa also endorsed meeting clients where they are while she helps them make meaning of their experiences with hearing voices. She said,

As far as meaning making, it's mostly just been discussing what significance the voices have for each patient. I've had patients who really enjoy their voices and they don't want to take medication to subdue them. And it kind of ties back to your last question about strength space. That's totally their choice. So I'm not going to emphasize, 'Hey, you need to take your medication because that would be the best option for you.' It's more-so talking about the pros and cons. If they don't find their voices to be harmful, then that's their choice and they have the right to make that decision. So just discussing, how helpful are they? Are they not helpful? What significance do they have to you? How are they impacting your day-to-day life? How have they impacted you in the past? Exploring things like that with them.

Amy agreed about meeting clients where they are, incorporating values when indicated, and empowering clients to collaborate in treatment. She stated that she wants to empower clients to feel like the process is collaborative and have some buy-in and belief in themselves to be able to make changes. At her internship site, she noted that she learns about clients' values during the initial psychosocial assessments that she conducts before beginning counseling with them. She also noted that with auditory verbal hallucinations, "it can be easy to get stuck on them as a barrier, or have the goal of treatment being symptom reduction." She said that she instead shifts her approach to, "How can we work with you as a whole person who hears voices?"

Elizabeth, working in an acute inpatient unit, noted that the extent to which she can help clients make meaning of their experiences is somewhat limited and that "I try to weave that in," but it depends due to clients' stays on the unit being transitional. When she has been able to work in meaning-making with clients even in a short time frame, she described this approach as, "I try to really meet them where they're at and individualize it, find what they can do, try to help support them in a way that they can reach recovery from their own strengths." Finally, Alisha noted that she takes a degree of caution regarding meaning-making and emphasized the client's interpretation of an experience as being more important than the therapist's. She cautioned clinicians to not project their own values on to clients' experiences:

> I feel like with something like that, you have to be careful because I can't make meaning of it. The client has to make meaning of it if they choose to make meaning of it. So I'll try to facilitate that discussion. You know, 'How does that make you feel? What does this mean to you? What do you make, where do you want to go?' You know, I'll never with meaning-making, I'll never try to, you know, put on my views or my perspectives on the client, but really encourage them to make sense of what that means to them, because I feel like that can be pretty impressive.

Belief in Recovery

Towards the end of the interview, clinicians were open-endedly asked to talk about the potential for recovery and what they believe recovery looks like for people who hear voices. Overwhelmingly, participants responded with answers that demonstrate a belief that recovery, at least in some way, is possible for clients with these experiences. Definitions of recovery differed among respondents' answers, but some themes emerged across interviews, including the definition of "recovery" being individualized and often non-linear; that recovery is possible but may not necessarily include eliminating voices; and that recovery involves self-advocacy and social supports.

"Recovery" is Individualized and Often Non-Linear

When asked about their thoughts on what recovery looks like for people who hear voices, participants overwhelmingly agreed that defining "recovery" is different for each client. As Karen said, "It's really about seeing success from their eyes." Alisha agreed, saying "Recovery looks the way they want it to look. It's not what I want it to look like." Rachel noted that "recovery" has become an overused term in the clinical literature and challenged professionals to consider that relying on a singular definition of this term can leave clients behind, as it does not account for individual differences. She noted that recovery should be conceptualized as "a personal definition that everyone can achieve." Marissa agreed that recovery is individualized and looks different for everyone and noted that "The difference may be in the way we conceptualize recovery. That's something that needs to be patient-centered." She succinctly worded her thoughts by saying, "It is different for every person and I think that it is up to every patient to determine for themselves."

Marissa also highlighted the importance of acknowledging recovery is often not a linear process. She shared her experience with normalizing non-linear recovery for clients and stated:

> One of the things we tell patients a lot is that it's not a linear process… and it can, it can take a while and that's okay. And sometimes you may experience an increase in the frequency in which you hear voices or their volume and or their

intensity, but also normalizing that and explaining, that's okay. And that it's part

of the recovery process.

Jacob agreed that definitions of recovery can differ for each client and noted that some of

these experiential differences may be related to the severity of psychotic symptoms. He

said:

> I think it's going to vary. I think for the more mild versions that might be living a
>
> normal life, you know, taking their medications, maybe they're not going to have
>
> a great family, but they're going to have some social connections. They're going
>
> to be able to maintain a job. They're going to have insight and be able to
>
> communicate. And as it gets more severe, I think we're talking more along the
>
> lines of being able to contact somebody when they're struggling or being aware
>
> that they're struggling. Even if they can't maintain work, and being able to be
>
> semi-independent, not necessarily being fully independent, but at least being
>
> semi-independent."

Recovery is Possible but May Not Involve Eliminating Voices

In addition to sharing beliefs that recovery was possible and often individualized,

many participants pointed out that these individual definitions of recovery do not always

involve a complete elimination of voices. Sarah described how clients may learn to view

their voices as a manageable experience, and stated that "for some, recovery is learning to

live with them and not let it influence your actions in a negative way." Nicholas agreed

that the individual definitions of recovery may involve learning to manage, rather than

eliminate, voices. He said:

If the term recovery is not experiencing hallucinations, without proper

management, is low. However, if the term recovery is based on just, you know,

symptom management, and achieving goals, and using strengths, that kind of

thing, I feel like it is a lot higher because you're not focusing on the lack of

something, right. And that we're not focusing on the lack of hallucinations, we're

focusing on more of what they want to accomplish.

Alisha also highlighted that recovery can involve learning to manage rather than eliminate voices. She stated:

Recovery is for someone, you know, still hearing the voices, but still managing to

thrive, still managing to have a quality of life. So managing that personal life. So

managing work, so managing to go to school, hey, that's recovery. It may not

always be completely getting rid of the voices, or the command hallucinations, if

that is what someone's recovery goal is, then that is fine.

Finally, Karen agreed that defining recovery may involve managing, rather than eliminating, the experience of hearing voices. She said, "I think recovery is about figuring out how to manage the cards you're dealt... and finding resilience in the midst of the game that you have to play."

Recovery Involves Self-Advocacy and Social Supports

As participants described their perspectives on recovery for people who hear voices, some clinicians included important factors that they believed to be essential for success. Some of the most frequently mentioned factors included clients' abilities to advocate for themselves and their needs, and the inclusion of social support in their environments. Regarding the importance of both self-advocacy and support, Karen shared,

> So we hear voices. Sometimes they're scary voices. Sometimes they're not scary voices. How can you take control of your life and test those voices? So is there someone in your life that you can ask, 'Did you hear that?' and trust that they're actually going to tell you the truth. They're not gonna play games with you or whatever. How can you use your treatment team to do that? If you choose to use medication, how does that work for you? How can we learn how to communicate with whoever's prescribing that medicine for you so that when you're entering maybe a more stressful season of your life, either for good reasons or bad, and you're like, man the voices are really ramping up. How do you communicate that to your helpers? That's recovery in my book.

She continued by further emphasizing the importance of a strong support network:

> It's a systemic thing. It's working with the rest of the family, of, you know, 'This is how we know when Bob is doing poorly. And this is how we know when Bob's doing well. This is how you can support Bob. When he asks you, if you hear what he hears something, be truthful with him.'

Lisa also emphasized the importance of clients advocating for themselves in their recovery, which includes knowing how to utilize their treatment team. She said,

> I think it will have a lot to do with medication adherence and sort of an acceptance around needing that additional support, or like just close collaboration with a psychiatrist so that if they don't need that support anymore, they do that safely. I think recovery...means...advocating for themselves as far as like what

they need. So if they're having an episode where they're feeling debilitated or they can't function or they're too distracted or whatever, they use the systems that are in place like FMLA or PTO to get some respite or mental health days to take care of those things.

Summary

The results from participant interviews provided insight into clinicians' experiences working with people who hear voices across multiple clinical settings, levels of experience, and experiences in education and training. The resulting themes from the data were outlined to reflect the interview protocol and the presenting research questions. The following chapter will be conclusions and discussion, which will include the final steps of Aspers' (2004) analytic procedure, including describing unintended consequences in the data, and relating the results to the existing literature. Answers to the research questions proposed by this study will clearly be addressed. In addition to this synthesis, limitations as well as implications for research, practice, training and education, and advocacy will be discussed.

CHAPTER V

DISCUSSION

This study aimed to learn about practitioners' experiences and perceptions of working with people who hear voices. In addition to asking open-ended questions about participants' experiences with clinical work in this area, I asked them if they had familiarity with people who are considered healthy voice-hearers who hear voices but do not experience significant distress. Additionally, I asked participants about their experiences in their doctoral programs regarding preparation for working with people who hear voices, as well as any training or education they may have received on positive psychology. I asked respondents to describe any elements of positive psychology that they use in their clinical work. Further, I inquired about participants' familiarity with critical theory, and described this theory as guiding my study. Finally, I asked the clinicians who were interviewed to discuss their beliefs about the potential for recovery for people who hear voices.

The first part of this final chapter outlines each of the above research questions and discusses the results from the interviews and how they address each question. To complete the final steps of Aspers' (2004) procedure for analysis, I discuss any unintended consequences that were revealed through analyzing interviews and relate the

152

results to the existing literature that was reviewed in Chapter II of this book. Next, I reveal limitations that were identified in the present study. Finally, this chapter concludes with implications across multiple domains (e.g., research, practice, training and education, and advocacy) so that readers receive a clear message about how they can use the results of this study in their own areas of interest.

Conclusions and Discussion across Research Questions

In the first segment of this chapter, I provide an outline of each research question and discuss the findings from my study as they relate to and address each question. Throughout this section, I include any unintended consequences that were revealed through analysis and synthesize the findings with the current relevant literature in the field. Throughout this Chapter, participants from clinical psychology programs may also be referred to as "clinical participants," "clinical practitioners," "clinicians from clinical programs," or "clinicians from clinical backgrounds," and participants from counseling psychology programs may also be referred to as "counseling participants," "counseling practitioners," "clinicians from counseling programs," or "clinicians from counseling backgrounds."

Research Question: Populations that Are Typically Worked with

The clinicians who were interviewed reported working in a variety of clinical settings in their past and present roles. The majority of the participants who were interviewed reported working in an inpatient hospital setting, including general hospitals, VA hospitals, state hospitals, and psychiatric inpatient facilities. Additionally, some participants who worked at non-hospital locations reported prior work in these settings. Many of the participants appeared to be eager to share an overview of some of their prior work settings, whether they were practicum or internship placements or different job sites. Although respondents were not specifically asked to share their previous work settings, many of them offered this information, and each of them reported a history of working in different areas. This information produced an unintended consequence, as it was not part of the interview protocol, but provided me with some valuable insight upon analysis. Even though I only asked participants about their present work sites, the fact that many of them shared previous experiences illuminates how valuable working in different settings can be for clinicians. Their varied clinical experiences suggest that clients who hear voices may present in any clinical setting and are not exclusively found in inpatient settings for acute psychosis as some people might believe.

Research Question: Therapeutic Approach to Working with People who Hear Voices

The clinicians who were interviewed endorsed using primary therapeutic approaches such as CBT, DBT, ACT, psychodynamic, person-centered, recovery-oriented, and illness management and recovery. Despite the differences expressed in their therapeutic orientations, participants identified the therapeutic alliance as being essential to successful work with clients, including those who hear voices. The therapeutic alliance is considered one of the core common factors in successful therapy, regardless of therapists' specific orientations or interventions (Wampold & Imel, 2015), and participants in this study echoed this understanding. The finding that the therapeutic alliance was important to practitioners from this study relates to findings by Jones et al. (2019), who found the therapeutic alliance to be a core theme among clinicians who were asked about their experiences of optimal client engagement. In the present study, both validation and the process of "joining with" clients were shared as techniques that clinicians use to strengthen the therapeutic bond and build rapport and trust with a client.

This finding is similar to the study by Larsson et al. (2012), where psychologists

constructed their experiences working with people with psychosis in a relational way,

including relating to and normalizing the experience. However, Larsson et al. (2012) only

sampled counseling psychologists, and the therapeutic relationship was shared as

important by clinicians from both counseling and clinical programs in my study.

Many participants described their experiences with navigating the clinical

environments in which they work in the context of the medical model. Emergent across

responses was advocacy of a combined approach that includes psychotherapy, social and

community support, and sometimes medication when indicated and accepted by the

client. These findings align with the biopsychosocial approach advocated by NICE

(2014) for work with people with psychosis, and also support Carter and colleagues'

(2017) results that found clinicians support a combination of psychosocial and

pharmacologic treatment. An emphasis on the importance of psychotherapy as an

alternative, or in conjunction with medication, was found in multiple interviews. Two

counseling psychologists provided a cautionary word about the field moving toward

strictly using protocols and other medical model approaches. Deborah remarked that

psychiatry is not akin to a pharmaceutical, and Adam shared his experience in a hospital

setting, where physicians make primary decisions and "psychotherapy is an adjunct"

instead of a primary treatment. Although I anticipated that I would find some skepticism

towards the medical model from counseling practitioners, I was surprised to find that

multiple clinical participants also shared a cautionary word on the topic. Several agreed

that medication should not be the sole component of a client's treatment plan, and also acknowledged some of the shortcomings of medication. As Rachel noted, taking antipsychotic medication does not guarantee a complete elimination of voices. Engaging in psychotherapy in conjunction with medication can help clients manage their experiences.

Research Question: Feelings and Biases about People who Hear Voices

Participants in this study were asked to open-endedly describe their feelings on working with people who hear voices. Participants overwhelmingly reported favorable views on this population, which was somewhat expected due to selection bias in the sample. One common element across interview responses involved a normalized view of hearing voices. Hearing voices may be viewed as any other symptom that a client presents with, so this experience is not treated by practitioners as particularly abnormal or shameful. Clinicians described normalizing the experience for clients, which may include validation and maintaining a clinical view that anyone may be susceptible to these experiences. As Rachel and Deborah described their perspectives on this possibility, anyone may be prone to having these experiences under different circumstances. During the interviews, this topic provided a helpful transition into the later questions that focus on healthy voice-hearers and clinicians' experiences and beliefs about people who hear voices but do not otherwise experience distress.

Although all the practitioners that I interviewed expressed enthusiasm or interest in working with people who hear voices, many also acknowledged that there is at least some level of challenge in working with this population. The sometimes slow rate of client progress and the recursive nature of recovery were cited as reasons for feeling frustrations as a clinician. However, participants who acknowledged this challenge also called the work with these clients "stressful, yet rewarding," and expressed a sense of satisfaction for working with clients who hear voices. Clinicians also spoke about their willingness to adjust their expectations in order to best work with clients based on where they are in treatment. This theme also emerged when speaking with participants about how they may help clients make meaning of their experiences and is further detailed in a later part of this chapter as part of the discussion on positive psychology questions.

Clinicians were also asked to describe the role of bias in working with these clients. Interestingly, participants were reluctant to disclose current personal biases and insisted that they enjoyed their work. When I asked this question, I had expected more honest disclosure of biases and dialogue about how all people have at least some form of implicit bias, even with all our training and exposure to diverse populations and experiences. Some participants were willing to speak about biases they held about people with psychosis or SMI clients prior to engaging in this work but did not speak about presently held biases. Participants' inabilities to disclose present biases may align with Gaertner and Dovidio's (1986) work on implicit bias and aversive racism. This work reveals that people may not demonstrate explicitly racist behavior or be aware of holding racist views, but have subconscious, implicit negative views of people who belong to different groups or identities. Although it is important to consider the role of implicit bias in working with diverse clients, it is possible that clinicians truly do possess fewer overall biases than the general population. As a study by Stull et al. (2013) found, mental health practitioners were found to hold positive explicit and implicit views towards people with mental illnesses. As the researchers of that study noted, these findings were consistent with Allport's (1954) contact hypothesis, which holds that intergroup contact under appropriate conditions can reduce prejudice between groups. When applied to clinicians, this hypothesis suggests that exposure to people with mental illnesses can reduce biases. Although Stull et al.'s (2013) study investigated practitioner bias, there appears to be sparse literature that focuses on biases towards people who hear voices or experience psychosis. Hansson et al. (2013) surveyed mental health practitioners about their attitudes towards clients and found that clinicians working with people with psychosis had the most negative attitudes of all surveyed clinicians. However, implicit bias was not measured here, and the study relied on self-report. Given these limitations, I was unable to identify many studies that focused on or meaningfully included an examination of practitioners' biases towards people with psychosis or people who hear voices. With the results of my present study, I wonder if a reason that this literature is sparse is because clinicians have a difficult time recognizing or admitting current bias in any form.

Clinicians were able, however, to identify the biases of other practitioners in the mental health field. They spoke about interns, co-workers, or professionals in other departments (e.g., physicians, nurses) as having biases about people who present with psychotic symptoms, including auditory verbal hallucinations. Several participants acknowledged the stigma that is experienced by many people with psychosis or who hear voices and shared their perceptions of other practitioners' biases or negative attitudes. A consideration to make from this finding is that mental health practitioners may have very different views and biases towards clients depending on the acuity and severity of their presenting symptoms. Mental health workers (e.g., counselors, social workers, nurses, psychiatrists) may have a limited perception on what the experience of hearing voices looks like based on the exposure to clients in their clinical settings. Although participants in the present study could not identify present biases, it is encouraging that they

acknowledged the barriers that stigma can place on clients' wellbeing and treatment. As

Yennari (2011) found clients to report that they felt a loss of freedom and control over

treatment when providers were perceived as uncaring and not taking them seriously,

several participants in the present study acknowledged that clients are aware of and

negatively impacted by practitioners with negative attitudes towards their experiences.

Research Question: Familiarity with Critical Theory

"Critical theory" as a term was unfamiliar to everyone who was interviewed,

however, many of the participants endorsed some familiarity with the concept once a

definition was provided. The lack of identification with this theory should perhaps not

have been surprising, as critical theory has mainly been used as a guiding framework in

scholarly discussions rather than in empirical studies that explore the experiences of SMI

clients. Psychologists were more likely to express lack of familiarity, and state that the

emerging literature is changing from when they were receiving their education. Prior to

conducting interviews, I wondered if current or very recent students (e.g., predoctoral or

postdoctoral interns) would be more familiar with the term than psychologists who had

been practicing for several years due to the recency of the theory appearing in literature

(Creswell, 2013). Although Alisha, a postdoctoral fellow was close to identifying the

concept, Deborah, a psychologist who has been practicing for years, also came close with

identifying critical race theory. There did not appear to be much difference among current

titles (e.g., intern, postdoc, psychologist) regarding the ability to identify the term or

mention related concepts, as no one had heard of critical theory by name. Most

participants stated an understanding and appreciation of the core components of recognizing oppressive factors and empowering marginalized people once the term was explained. This recognition by many participants is encouraging, as it shows that many clinicians have an awareness of societal factors that influence their clients' experiences and acknowledge the role that power and oppression have in the experiences of marginalized groups (Merriman, 2009).

Research Question: Healthy Voice-Hearers

When asked about healthy voice-hearers, clinicians had not heard of the term as it is presented in the literature (Baumeister et al., 2017). This was a somewhat expected finding, as healthy voice-hearers have only sparsely and recently been studied and discussed in academic journals, and may not at all be reviewed in coursework, because by definition they do not meet criteria for a mental illness. Although no one recognized the term healthy voice-hearers, many respondents were familiar with people who fell into or near that category. Some participants provided personal examples of people from past or present personal relationships who have heard voices without functional impairment. Elizabeth's example about her husband changing the content of his voices' messages through kindly responding to them reflects Baumeister and colleagues' (2017) findings that positive messages, including advice-giving, may be found more in healthy voice-hearers than in clinical voice-hearers.

Even if participants did not disclose personal relationships with healthy voice-hearers, many acknowledged that multicultural factors are taken into account when they conceptualize clients' experiences. For example, William, Bruce, and Sarah all described how hearing voices may be considered a religious or important familial experience in Latinx or Hispanic cultures. Sociocultural factors were accounted for by participants as well. Rachel's case vignette involved a client who heard voices that he believed to be former fellow gang members. Bruce accounted for cultural, religious, and criminogenic factors as well when conceptualizing the client who began committing crimes to regain a sense of power over the voices, as he believed that his personal sense of power had been stolen.

Several participants brought up the Hearing Voices Network when they were asked about healthy voice-hearers. One of the most educational pieces of conducting this study for me was learning from participants about the Hearing Voices Network, the global peer support community for people who hear voices that I had somehow missed during my initial research. I wondered if by limiting my reading selections to peer-reviewed studies in academic journals, I perhaps overlooked additional sources of information such as the Hearing Voices Network. I was intrigued to hear from my participants about their experiences with this community; several clinicians had facilitated groups for this network and likened it to a social justice movement or a new framework for understanding voices. The most similar overlap I found with my literature review and the Hearing Voices Network are peer support treatments for psychosis. As many of the activities that this network participates in are led and attended by people who hear voices, Hearing Voices Network may meet Chien's (2019) definitional criteria of a peer support treatment, featuring peers with similar difficulties who support one another. However, one key difference here is that members of the Hearing Voices Network may not view hearing voices as being problematic; they normalize the experience and in some cases reject diagnoses or pathologizing these experiences. This group may meet the underlying assumption of the peer support approach, which is that people who share similar experiences are considered more equal in the relationship than clients and therapists in their respective therapeutic relationship roles (Dennis, 2003).

Research Question: Doctoral Education and Training

Clinicians who were interviewed spoke about their experiences not only working with people who hear voices, but also about any education and training they received with this population during their doctoral programs. As I analyzed the data from this study, I realized that my expectations were biased towards expecting people from clinical psychology programs to have more significant training in working with people with psychosis than they reported. Although I found that many clinical practitioners reported receiving some coursework in working with clients with psychosis, I was surprised to find that clinical participants reported varied exposure to this population in their training. Although several clinical practitioners reported that they received coursework that was specific to psychopathology, SMI clients, or psychosis, a greater number reported only partially receiving this type of formal education. Participants who reported this partial exposure to psychosis in their coursework spoke about having a class on assessment or the DSM, where screening for psychotic disorders was mentioned but not explored in depth. Additionally, other participants reported little to no coursework that featured education on SMI or psychosis. I was surprised that this type of education was less reported than I had expected, due to the historical adherence to the medical model in clinical psychology (Seligman, 2002; Yip, 2005). Although I was surprised by this finding, it resembles a result from a study by Jones et al. (2019), who found that clinicians felt underprepared for working with people with psychosis due to lack of psychosis-specific education in school. Jones and others' (2019) study included a sample of a wider range of mental health practitioners that was not limited to psychologists, but this finding still highlights a lack of psychosis-specific training across programs. In the present study, participants from counseling psychology programs did not report much formal education or training about psychosis; two participants recalled a brief overview of psychotic disorders in a diagnostic course, whereas the two others recalled "no formal training" in this area. This result was somewhat expected, due to counseling psychology's criticism of the medical model and historical tendency to work with more "healthy" populations or in vocational guidance roles (Delgado-Romero et al., 2012). Additionally, some participants mentioned receiving more education related to psychosis in their Master's programs than they did in their doctoral studies. Participants who spoke about their predoctoral graduate studies spoke about them dismissively and as an afterthought, so this may be considered an unintended consequence revealed through participants' words that they may not have considered as significant to their response at the time of the interview. Although they viewed the experiences that they described receiving in their Master's programs as important to their training if it involved exposure to psychosis, they did not spend time elaborating. Rather, they focused the majority of their responses to describing their lack of this type of education in their doctoral programs.

Participants across disciplines shared a common experience of receiving more exposure to psychosis during their practicum experiences than they did in their academic classes. As with my surprise that clinical practitioners received less education on psychosis than I expected, I was also initially not expecting these clinicians to report that their education came mainly from practica. However, after speaking with multiple participants, I began to realize that this finding made sense; as with any discipline, many people learn better from "hands-on" practice than they do from reading books and having discussions with colleagues. As illustrated by the case vignettes each participant shared with me, each client is unique and complex. In a sense, all the academic reading in the world cannot rival meeting and working with a real client and their many stories, experiences, beliefs, and intersecting identities. Still though, there may be more room for both clinical and counseling programs to incorporate lessons that prepare students to work with people who hear voices or experience psychosis. This topic is further detailed in the "implications" section of this chapter.

Research Question: Familiarity with and Use of Positive Psychology

Clinicians who were interviewed were asked to describe their familiarity with positive psychology. They were also prompted to speak about any education they received on this topic in their doctoral programs, as well as if and how they incorporate positive psychology into their client interventions, specifically when working with people who hear voices. Counseling practitioners endorsed more familiarity with the term "positive psychology" than did clinical participants, and they tended to report that they received some formal education in this area. Even for counseling clinicians who did not recall receiving structured coursework on positive psychology, they each were able to identify major tenets of the movement. This finding supports the foundational research that acknowledges a meaningful overlap between counseling and positive psychology in its core principles, including a focus on client strengths, assets, and potentialities (APA, 1999; Gelso & Fretz, 2001; Savickas, 2003).

Although participants from counseling psychology backgrounds endorsed familiarity with positive psychology in the academic sense, I was surprised to find that both clinical and counseling practitioners identified that they used elements of positive

psychology in their interventions with clients who hear voices. Regardless of which

primary therapeutic modality clinicians identified using, they each were able to identify

using some intervention that relates to positive psychology. Therapists identified their

primary therapeutic approaches in multiple ways, including ACT, DBT, CBT, person-

centered, recovery-oriented, and insight-oriented treatments. Incorporating client values

and strengths was something that many participants reported using in their work with

people who hear voices. Although not all participants may have considered their

treatment approaches as being related to positive psychology prior to these interviews,

after speaking with them, it was evident that they use interventions that may be

considered under the positive psychology umbrella. As Drvaric et al. (2015) define

positive psychology interventions, many clinicians who were interviewed endorsed using

therapeutic treatments that facilitate the effective use of strengths to solve problems and

build resilience. The fact that multiple clinicians from diverse backgrounds and with

varied therapeutic orientations agreed on using positive psychology interventions

demonstrates the versatility and universality of such methods.

When asked if and how they help clients make meaning of their experiences,

many clinicians agreed that they did, and mentioned that they try to meet clients where

they are. Much like the framework for helping people cope with psychosis proposed by

Roe et al. (2006) that involves proactive coping, participants in the present study

identified ways to help clients identify what activities are meaningful to them. This

finding also connects with a later section of the discussion that focuses on belief in

recovery. Practitioners identified that recovery is often individualized and may involve improving daily functioning and learning to use one's support system, which highlights an example of meeting clients where they are. Acknowledging that each client is unique, and everyone presents with different levels of functioning or impairment, in order to work with a client towards recovery, therapists take these individual factors into account when planning treatment and engaging in this work. Helping clients make meaning of their experiences can connect with positive psychology (Roe et al., 2006), but also can be understood in the context of existential psychotherapy. Yalom (1980) considered "meaning-in-life" to be a core psychological construct, and noted in his existential psychotherapy text, "The human being seems to require meaning. To live without meaning, goals, values, or ideals, seems to provoke considerable distress." Clinicians have the potential to help clients work through feelings of meaningless by learning about the clients' beliefs and the importance of meaning in their lives (Yalom, 1980). Although the participants in the present study may not have identified positive nor existential psychology as their primary therapeutic approaches, many of them endorsed meaning-making as a part of their treatment for clients hearing voices.

Research Question: Beliefs about Recovery for People who Hear Voices

Finally, participants were asked to share their beliefs about the potential for recovery for people who hear voices. Participants all endorsed a belief that some sort of recovery is possible for clients with these experiences. Although this finding was encouraging and uplifting, I admit that I was somewhat surprised that no one expressed a view that recovery was impossible or even unlikely. However, there was some form of sample bias with this study, as the participants who agreed to complete the interviews were likely to be interested in clients who experience psychosis. This bias is further described in the limitations section of this chapter.

A key commonality that participants shared, in addition to believing recovery is possible, is that "recovery" is an individualized definition for each client and is oftentimes non-linear. Although not all clinicians endorsed familiarity with positive psychology by definition, nearly everyone described recovery as being personal. Many participants noted that this personal definition of recovery may involve clients functioning well in multiple areas of their lives, even if they were still experiencing voices. This perspective that was shared by many participants echoes a core belief of positive psychology, in that people have the potential to flourish even while continuing to experience symptoms including psychosis (Slade, 2010). Additionally, this finding is similar to the definition of recovery presented by Meyer et al. (2012), in identifying that recovery is different for each client and meaningfully defined on an individual basis. Clinicians also pointed out that recovery is often non-linear, meaning that someone may experience fluctuations with factors such as the volume and intensity of voices, or have periods of time where the voices disappear then return. These same clinicians all agreed that they acknowledge this as an expected part of the recovery process and try to normalize these experiences with their clients so that they feel validated and not discouraged.

Recovery was also acknowledged as not necessarily involving a complete elimination of voices. Rather, clients may learn how to better manage their voices, whether that is through making meaning of their personal relationship with the voices, addressing them directly, tuning them out through music, quieting them with earplugs or medication, or any other methods that were not mentioned by participants. I welcomed

learning from different clinicians about some of the methods for voice management that

had worked for their clients and found that participants offered this information

throughout the interviews. Whereas some respondents verbalized their belief that

recovery may not involve eliminating voices when asked about recovery, they and other

participants also mentioned some of these various methods for voice management when

speaking about their clients during earlier interview questions. This tendency to speak

about client strategies for managing voices without specific prompting suggests that

clinicians can value symptom management rather than elimination. Considering my

research into the historical context and present tendency of clinical psychologists to

adhere to the medical model and push for "fixing" problematic symptoms (Yip, 2005), I

was surprised to find that both clinical and counseling practitioners did not push clients to

eliminate their voices or view them as necessarily negative or abnormal experiences.

Rather, this perspective aligns with positive psychology interventions, which tend to

focus more on proactive coping skills and making meaning rather than fully eliminating

voices (e.g., Boiler, 2013; Meyer et al., 2012; Schrank et al., 2016).

Two key factors were also identified by participants as being integral to recovery;

clients' ability to advocate for themselves, and their ability to access and utilize social

supports. These essential factors also can be considered as occurring together, not in

isolation. For example, when Karen shared her thoughts on successful recovery, she

emphasized the importance of a client knowing when and how to use their treatment

team, and when to ask for help. Being able to utilize a support system (e.g., caseworker,

psychiatrist, therapist, family members) inherently includes some self-advocacy, as asking for help is a powerful form of working to get one's needs met This finding that self-advocacy and utilizing supports are essential to recovery aligns with the indications for best outcomes for people with psychosis (Lehman et al., 2010; NICE, 2010) that includes a biopsychosocial approach of medication, psychotherapy, and social support. Clients who feel able to ask for what they need from the appropriate supports have better chances for their version of successful recovery, even if the definition of recovery is individualized and may involve learning to live with, rather than eliminate, the voices that they hear.

Limitations

There were several limitations present in this study, mainly involving the sampling methods. The sample of this study consisted of fourteen participants. The size of the sample was deliberately selected to be between twelve and fifteen participants, or until saturation was reached. Whereas the target sample size was met, the demographic sample of participants was not as heterogenous as desired. I aimed to meet with a diverse sample of participants with equal representation in terms of specialty (e.g., counseling or clinical psychology), gender, and racial and ethnic background. However, most participants were from clinical backgrounds, female, and White. Although I was able to speak with some participants from different racial backgrounds, most of the people that I spoke with identified as White or Caucasian, which may have limited the range of experiences I could have learned from a more diverse sample. Although I aimed to speak with more participants from a counseling psychology background, I was only able to meet with four participants with this training. Whereas the resulting sample provided me with more experiences from clinical psychology practitioners, this disparity in numbers of clinical and counseling psychologists appears to reflect differences in the psychologist population at large. According to a survey by the APA (APA, 2016), roughly half (45.1%) of licensed psychologists are clinical, with less than ten percent (9.4%) being counseling psychologists. Similarly, the predominantly female sample reflects the population of psychologists being comprised mostly of women (59.2% of psychologists identified as female, APA, 2016), and the predominantly White sample in this study reflects the racial demographics (87.8% of psychologists identified as white or Caucasian). Finally, another demographic disparity in this study involved the majority of participants working as psychologists ($n = 9$), with less participants working as predoctoral interns ($n = 3$) and postdoctoral fellows ($n = 2$).

One unique challenge that was presented during this study involved recruiting and interviewing participants during the COVID-19 global pandemic. The original interviewing method was planned to present prospective participants with the option of meeting in person for the interview or completing it remotely through Zoom. During this planning process, I had a preference in mind for face-to-face interviews, as these methods would allow me to observe body language and other nonverbal behavior more easily than using the virtual format. However, in-person interviews were not possible due to health risks brought on by the pandemic. Although I was able to adapt and potentially reach a wider audience of recruits virtually, I did not have the opportunity to meet people face-to-face and broaden my observations. My interviews were recorded via Zoom to later be transcribed, but this method introduced room for technological error. The interview with my final participant, Amy, was unfortunately not recorded due to these errors, and for her interview analysis I had to rely on notes that I had taken throughout the session using my interview protocol and shorthand notation. Because of this challenge, rich data in the form of direct quotations was lost for this participant.

Selection bias was also a factor to consider in the sample for this study. Because the selection criteria required participants to have worked with at least one client who experienced hearing voices, there is an assumption that participants have an interest in working with and speaking about this population. This is important to keep in mind when considering participants' reported lack of biases and optimistic views for recovery and wellbeing. Additionally, the sample was limited to psychologists and psychology trainees. This sample represents a limited selection of the larger population of mental health professionals, which can include people who work with clients who may be experiencing acute psychosis and be in crisis (e.g., social workers, psychiatric nurses, case managers). Many of the clients that participants spoke about for their case vignettes were people they worked with over weeks, months, or years. The length of these therapeutic relationships reflects that the clinicians had an opportunity to work with clients in-depth and get to understand their experiences with hearing voices, rather than stabilizing clients who were experiencing acute psychosis. Another important limitation of this study relates to this acknowledgement. Although this study focuses on learning from healthy voice-hearers and helping clients make meaning of their experiences with voices, these approaches may not be indicated for every client with these experiences. Many of the clients whose stories were shared during this study may be classified as closer to mild than to severe on the psychosis continuum (Baumeister et al., 2017). Clients who are experiencing acute psychotic episodes or who experience severe psychotic symptoms may require more intensive interventions that may involve hospitalization or medical interventions for stabilization. Acknowledging the differences that clients may have in terms of symptom severity is important when considering which treatment approaches are most appropriate for each person.

Implications

The following section of this paper is organized by types of implications that this study has for practical use by interested readers. These areas of interest include implications for future research, clinical practice, training and education, and advocacy. The aim of this portion of the chapter is to encourage readers to take with them some practical knowledge from this study and think about ways that they can make changes in their areas of influence that align with this study's core values.

Implications for Future Research

This study was unique in its sampling from both counseling and clinical psychologists, predoctoral, and postdoctoral interns, and its exploration of clinicians' experiences in working with people who hear voices, with healthy-voice-hearers, with positive psychology, critical theory, and their belief in recovery for people who hear voices. Participants also provided insight about their training programs and how they learned (or did not learn) about topics such as positive psychology, psychosis, and critical theory. As the extant literature on clinician's perspectives of people with psychosis is limited, the literature on clinicians' perspectives of people who are healthy voice-hearers is even more sparse. This work provides a good starting point for future research that could build from the lessons found here.

Prospective researchers could expand on and improve the present study by addressing some of the limitations that were identified. One key area for improvement is the sample of participants who may be interviewed in a future study. A more racially diverse sample of practitioners may be reached by making some changes to the recruitment process. The questions that the researcher plans to ask, and the resulting interview protocol may be tailored to align with interests or issues experienced by clinicians of Color. The interview protocol for such a study may be developed by a more racially diverse team of researchers to represent the needs of a diverse sample of participants more accurately. Additionally, a more diverse sample in terms of training background (e.g., counseling or clinical) and job title (e.g., psychologist, predoctoral or postdoctoral intern) may be recruited by targeting the interview protocol to speak about experiences specific to these educational or present job factors. Techniques for recruiting can also be improved upon by increasing outreach to different APA divisions or through utilizing researchers' other professional networks. Finally, interviews may be conducted in person to fully capture participants' reactions and responses, including nonverbal behaviors.

An area for future research that I propose based on some of my more surprising findings focuses on clinicians' biases, including an unwillingness or inability to acknowledge present biases. The Implicit Association Test (Greenwald et al., 1998) or a similarly designed implicit bias test could include people with psychosis or people who hear voices as a category. This inclusion would not only identify them as a marginalized population, but also allow people (clinicians included) to test for biases they may have learned through life experience and interactions of which they may not be aware. Researchers could utilize other methods of testing biases to further explore this area with clinicians regarding people who hear voices.

Another somewhat surprising finding from this study provides more opportunities for future research to build off this work. Many participants shared examples of working with (in clinical or personal life) people who hear voices but otherwise function well in daily life. This finding suggests that healthy voice-hearers may be more common than expected or reported. As the research with healthy voice hearers is relatively new and therefore somewhat limited, additional research can be done in this area. Prospective researchers could begin this work by sampling either people who hear voices, or clinicians who have worked with healthy voice-hearers. Although this study used an adequate sample size for its qualitative methodology, larger-scale research could be conducted with a larger sample size using quantitative methods. A survey that asks about experiences with hearing voices and how these experiences are managed or conceptualized could highlight the prevalence of healthy-voice-hearers as well as identify common factors that people with these experiences may share.

Another area of research that could be expanded upon from this study is the use of positive psychology interventions for hearing voices. As I identified in the literature review section of this paper, there is already promising evidence for positive psychology interventions for people with psychosis. However, this study adds an element of universality to this literature, as participants endorsed using various primary treatment approaches, none of which was positive psychology. Still, everyone who was interviewed reported using at least some elements of positive psychology (e.g., using client's strengths, helping them make meaning of their experiences) in their clinical work. Although they may not have identified themselves as using positive psychology without these interview questions, many of them are still influenced in some way by this approach. Additional research could involve interviewing clinicians across varied

therapeutic orientations (e.g., CBT, psychodynamic, person-centered) and investigating

the prevalence of positive psychology interventions or approaches that are used in their

work, even if they are called by a different name. Finally, the definition of clinicians as

participants can be expanded to include people who engage in work in inpatient hospital

settings and regularly see clients who are experiencing crises, including acute psychosis.

Speaking to practitioners who work in different settings may expand the research on

clinicians' views of clients who hear voices and their work with them.

Implications for Clinical Practice

Clinicians from different educational backgrounds can all take away some

applicable lessons from this study to incorporate into their clinical work. An important

starting point for applying this knowledge can be honestly examining personal biases.

While acknowledging the details of prior biases and noting progress in working through

these can be meaningful, each clinician can also realize that many biases are rooted in our

upbringings and societal standards, and we each hold at least some form of bias. Thus,

examining present biases can provide insight into how we each view people who hold

different identities. These biases may be considered implicit biases, which are shaped by

experience and learned associations between certain qualities and social categories. The

Implicit Association Test, also known as the Harvard Implicit Bias Test (Greenwald,

McGhee, & Schwartz, 1998) is available online, and can reveal to test-takers the degrees

to which we hold implicit biases towards groups of people including women, people of

color, people of size, people who identify as gay, people with disabilities, and older

people. Although examining these biases can help practitioners work with all clients by being aware of learned stereotypes and avoiding microaggressions, this work can also be helpful when working with people who hear voices. As mentioned above in the implications for research section of this chapter, people with psychosis and psychosis-related symptoms may be considered a marginalized population in regards to the stigma they experience from society. The APA Multicultural Guidelines (APA, 2017) provide guidance for examining how contexts of identities can inform biases, encouraging psychologists to not only consider clients' intersecting identities, but also examine their own. Through processing how a clinician's various identities interact with those of their clients, they can expand their empathy and understanding of a client's experience, including the impact that sociocultural and structural forces have on them (APA, 2017).

Many of the clinicians who were interviewed demonstrated an interest in working with people who hear voices, helped validate and normalize experiences for their clients, and were aware of people who hear voices and view them as positive or personally meaningful. Since there was some selection bias in this study because of participants choosing to take part in this research, it is not fair to assume that all clinicians express the same views. With this realization in mind, all clinicians who come across this study may learn from its participants and honestly reflect about how they conceptualize and treat clients who hear voices. Taking cultural and other contextual factors into consideration is important for clinical work with all people and should be applied to clients' experiences of hearing voices as well. Since some level of frustration or challenge is often experienced when working with clients with psychosis, therapists should be prepared to process these feelings in the appropriate format (e.g., with a supervisor, through journaling, or consultation with another clinician). Clinicians can benefit from continuing education and may seek out additional training specific to working with people who hear voices. They can also benefit from expanding their framework for understanding the experiences of marginalized populations, including people with psychosis, by learning more about critical theory. In addition to conducting their own research by reviewing available literature (e.g., Creswell, 2013), therapists can seek out workshops, webinars, or forums that involve critical theory.

Additionally, practitioners from all disciplines can learn from positive psychology and consider how they may use clients' strengths in their work, as well as help clients make meaning of their experiences. They may start this process by reviewing available resources to familiarize themselves with the efficacy of positive psychotherapy interventions (e.g., a meta-analysis by Bolier et al., 2013), and learning about specific interventions. For example, clinicians could learn about using WELLFOCUS positive psychotherapy (Schrank et al., 2016), helping clients process significant life events through thinking, writing, and talking (Lyubomirsky et al., 2006) or boosting resilience while building strengths (Drvaric et al., 2015). Additionally, clinicians could try working with a client to identify areas that they believe are strengths. If clients struggle to come up with strengths, the clinician may identify some (e.g., "You've made a point of coming to therapy consistently and on time for x weeks, so you are able to follow through on commitments"). The therapist can then work these strengths into the client's treatment plan. To help clients make meaning of their experiences, clinicians can begin by meeting the client where they are. Many of the participants in this study spoke about their willingness to work with clients at their level of functioning and readiness for change. Clinicians may learn from these participants and practice the same with their clients.

Working with clients at their level can also involve adjusting expectations, which may include viewing recovery as recursive and may include managing, rather than eliminating, voices. An additional consideration to make when considering positive psychology interventions is that the clinicians in this study endorsed a wide range of therapeutic approaches, so these interventions are versatile and can be incorporated into many different treatment modalities.

Finally, clinicians can take from this study two meaningful elements of client recovery: self-advocacy and utilizing social supports. The theme of self-advocacy may be viewed within the framework of critical theory, which acknowledges that practitioners have the ability not only to advocate on behalf of clients, but to empower them to advocate for themselves as well (Parker, 2015). Clinicians may begin to think about how they can empower their clients to advocate for themselves and their needs. This work may involve processing the therapeutic alliance with the client, and creating and reinforcing a safe, supportive space where the client is comfortable expressing their needs. Just as Alisha allowed her client to wear earphones during sessions to block the voices, clinicians may ask clients what can be helpful for them to feel most comfortable and willing to engage in sessions. Utilizing social supports was also found to be a meaningful theme in clinicians' perspectives of client recovery. This finding aligns with the biopsychosocial approach advocated by NICE (2010) and its social support component to factors for successful treatment outcomes. Therapists can also support their clients in utilizing their treatment team. Clients who have multiple healthcare workers (e.g., caseworker, psychiatrist) may benefit from processing and planning with the therapist to prepare for visits and be able to express their needs (e.g., verbalizing

medication side-effects or being honest about completing applications for benefits).
Clinicians can review with clients their social support network, which may include family
members, friends, co-workers, or peers through groups such as Hearing Voices Network
or any twelve-step program or other group, and work with them on how these
relationships are meaningful and beneficial to them.

Implications for Training and Education

The present study involved learning from psychologists (and people very near to
being psychologists) from both counseling and clinical psychology backgrounds.
Through my interviews with practitioners from both backgrounds, I learned some
valuable information about peoples' experiences with their education and training, and
how it prepared them (or did not) for working with people with psychosis as well as
incorporating a client's strengths into their clinical work. This section on training and
education implications provides key takeaways that may be implemented by both
counseling and clinical psychology doctoral training programs.

One area for growth that was identified when interviewing participants was that
there is room in doctoral programs for including lessons about who experience psychosis
or hear voices. Many clinical psychology doctoral programs include at least some
coursework that involves education on conceptualizing, diagnosing, and/or treating SMI
clients, including people who experience psychosis. Although the present study found
that most participants from clinical programs received at least some education on
psychosis, the quantity and depth of this education was less than expected. Counseling
psychology programs tend to emphasize some elements of positive psychology, such as
encouraging a holistic view of each client and utilizing a client's strengths in treatment

179

(APA, 1999; Gelso & Fretz, 2001; Savickas, 2003). Although counseling psychologists take pride in not overpathologizing clients from a deficit perspective, there is a missed opportunity for embracing a holistic, strengths-based approach while working with clients with psychosis or clients who hear voices. Both types of psychology programs may not provide adequate coursework in serious mental illness, including psychosis. Incorporating lessons on working with people with psychosis does not mean that counseling psychology programs need to abandon the values on which counseling psychology was formed. Instead of teaching courses using a deficits-based model, instructors can acknowledge problems and distress that many clients who hear voices experience, but also highlight ways to use clients' strengths in treatment, consider contextual factors in their conceptualization, and honor their perspectives on what hearing voices means to them. These lessons may be woven into the curricula of counseling psychology programs using the Model Training Program (Scheel et al., 2018). This program guides the development and maintenance of counseling psychology programs and highlights core values including growth towards full potential, holistic and contextual values, diversity and social justice values, and a communitarian perspective, and aligns with many of the values of positive psychology expressed by the Division 17 Section on Positive Psychology.

Both clinical and counseling psychology educators can also initiate conversations with students about examining their biases as clinicians as they prepare to enter work with diverse clients, including those who may experience symptoms of psychosis. Finally, instructors may consider engaging in discussions about healthy voice-hearers, and how each person who hears voices has a unique experience. A key lesson that may be taught here is that clinicians can strive to balance their clinical expertise in treatment planning with honoring client's preferences, perceptions, and beliefs, keeping in mind that not everyone who hears voices experiences dysfunction or distress. Finally, it was found that clinicians received more experience working with psychosis when working directly in the field rather than in the classroom. Just as Jones et al.'s (2019) study with mental health workers across training backgrounds found, even clinical psychologists in the present study reported that they felt underprepared for work with clients with psychosis based on their education alone. Further, many practitioners had to seek out experiences with this population on their own. Both types of doctoral programs could benefit students by incorporating more psychosis-specific lessons into their curricula. Additionally, doctoral programs could consider expanding the variety of clinical settings that students may select for practicum experiences, including more community mental health centers, hospitals, and forensic sites. Expanding students' exposure to different clinical settings and populations can enable future psychologists to gain broader experience and apply their field's core values to their work with diverse clients.

Doctoral programs that do not currently utilize a holistic approach can incorporate more education about contextual factors and multicultural variables into their lessons on everything from etiology to diagnosis to treatment, and more fully integrate these concepts into their lessons. Ideally, multicultural and contextual factors could be woven into the lessons in each course (e.g., when discussing case conceptualization or reviewing treatment planning), but a course that focuses on multicultural factors could be incorporated into a clinical program as well. Through including this type of education in classes, the holistic approach that is assumed by many counseling psychologists can be adopted by clinical programs as well. Additionally, providing students from both types of programs with education on systemic factors through a critical theory lens (Creswell, 2013) can enable them to see clients in the context of their environment, and as a whole person rather than maintaining a narrow focus on their diagnoses or presenting problems. Specifically, clinical psychology programs can incorporate critical theory lessons into pre-existing courses (e.g., qualitative research classes, or theory or philosophy classes), or develop new courses to present this material. Clinical programs can learn from some of counseling psychology's core values, including belief in social justice and advocacy (Packard, 2009) and incorporate social justice or policy classes into their curriculum.

Finally, doctoral programs can incorporate education about biases, including implicit biases, into their coursework. Just as current biases were not acknowledged in the present study, many clinicians and emerging clinicians may not be aware of implicit bias and could benefit personally and professionally from this type of education. Educators may facilitate this process by encouraging students to engage in reflective writing where they identify their social locations and identities of privilege and oppression. Students and educators may also complete the Implicit Association Test (Greenwald et al., 1998) and engage in meaningful dialogue about the formation and maintenance of implicit biases for multiple marginalized identities. Educators can then further elaborate on this conversation by including dialogue about how people who are classified as SMI or people who hear voices may be considered a marginalized population that experiences stigma and bias as well.

Implications for Advocacy

When considering implications from this study that may be applied across different spheres of influence, some suggestions are provided for people who want to advocate for people who hear voices and affect the way society views and treats people with these experiences. Readers who are interested in advocacy may begin by continuing to seek education on this topic. The literature review in this paper provides a starting point from which interested readers can search for articles that address topics of advocacy interest, including stigma, healthy voice-hearers, and critical theory. For people who are interested in challenging the way they think about and view things, readings on critical theory can be particularly enlightening. Creswell (2013), for example, provides an informative introduction to the topic as well as describes ways people may use this theory to guide advocacy. Because a core tenet of critical theory is empowering marginalized people to transcend societal constraints, reading more into this topic may inspire people to change their approach to their work. For example, anyone who works in the healthcare field (which may include mental health, but also medical practitioners) can start by recognizing the power differential inherent to all clinician-client relationships. Further research on stigma can include seeking out information about the experiences that people who experience acute psychosis may have, and how society may view these in a negative manner. Learning about how psychosis presents differently for different people can help people gain awareness of the diversity of experiences and the corresponding challenges. For example, an acute phase of psychosis may only reflect part of someone's experience and not include their experiences of maintenance throughout their lives.

Another avenue of research for advocates could involve reading more about the Hearing Voices Network (National Hearing Voices Network, 2021). Even if someone does not experience hearing voices or know anyone who does, interested people may browse the materials on this organization's website to familiarize themselves with preferred terminology (e.g., "hearing voices" rather than "auditory verbal hallucinations") and the core values shared by members. The organization also offers trainings that are suitable for not only people who hear voices or professionals, but also "anyone with an interest in this area." Some of these trainings include workshops and courses that can equip participants with the tools for starting a Hearing Voices group or gaining a deeper understanding of what it can mean to hear voices and how to support people with these experiences. Additional resources are listed on this website as well if people are curious to learn more from sources that are trusted and supported by people who share the experience of hearing voices.

Another important form of advocacy that readers can practice is listening to, validating, and otherwise supporting anyone who they know who hears voices. Readers who may have a family member, significant other, friend, or other close relationship with someone who shares that they hear voices can begin with nonjudgmental listening. Not all people who hear voices seek treatment or experience significant distress, and not all people who hear voices choose to share these experiences with others. Being supportive to people who share this information is important, but so is using nonjudgmental language across all settings. For example, eliminating words like "crazy" or "schizophrenic" or "psychotic" as a pejorative from one's vocabulary can seem subtle, but really be important in reducing stigma and normalizing experiences.

Readers who are interested in expanding their advocacy efforts to the societal level may consider ways that they can influence public policy. Individuals can begin by learning about the officials that are running for governmental positions at the local, state, and federal levels, and voting and promoting candidates who value mental health. Individuals can get involved in lobbying campaigns for areas that influence mental health services, such as increasing funding or introducing legislation that increases the visibility or provides equity to the SMI population. Interested readers may consider donating, fundraising, or volunteering to support mental health organizations (e.g., the National Alliance on Mental Illness; Mental Health America) or beginning grassroots campaigns to recruit other advocates and spread awareness of stigma and other barriers faced by these individuals and propose actionable changes.

Summary

This qualitative study was conducted in effort to learn more from practitioners from counseling and clinical backgrounds and to address some gaps in the literature on the topic of people who hear voices. This study provided an opportunity to learn from clinicians about their experiences and beliefs about working with people who hear voices; their therapeutic approach to working with this population; how their doctoral education and training prepared them for this work; their familiarity with healthy-voice-hearers, critical theory, and positive psychology; the extent to which positive psychology influences their work with this population; and their belief in recovery for people who hear voices and seek treatment. The development of this study and the interview protocol was guided by critical theory, and how people who hear voices may be viewed as a marginalized population within this context. The empirical phenomenological approach that was used for data analysis honored individual experiences that participants shared while looking for common themes among responses.

Clinicians' therapeutic approaches to working with people with psychosis varied, but they acknowledged the importance of the therapeutic alliance in treatment and expressed some skepticism towards the medical model. Their feelings about working with people who hear voices were generally positive, although they expressed some level of challenge in this work. Participants shared a normalized, rather than pathologized, view of hearing voices. Although they may have acknowledged prior personal biases in their work with this population, they denied present biases, but had observed biases from other mental health professionals. Most participants were unfamiliar with the term "critical theory," but many were familiar with related concepts. Similarly, clinicians were unfamiliar with the term "healthy voice-hearers," although many were familiar with the concept, and some spoke about their experiences with the Hearing Voices Network. Many participants acknowledged the importance of considering cultural factors when working with clients who hear voices. As they spoke about their doctoral training, participants revealed that they received more experience working with people with psychosis at their practicum sites than they did in the classroom. Several participants from clinical psychology programs indicated that they received some coursework in psychosis (and felt somewhat prepared to work with this population), but they reported less of this type of education than expected. Participants noted that their clinical experience with this population was often a choice that they had to seek out on their own. Participants with counseling psychology backgrounds frequently reported using a holistic approach to their clinical work and reported familiarity with positive psychology.

Regardless of their primary therapeutic approach, several participants reported emphasizing a client's strengths in treatment, and many believed that helping clients make meaning of their experiences involves meeting them where they are. Finally, as clinicians described their belief in the potential for recovery for people who hear voices, they agreed that recovery is possible, but different for each person and often non-linear. Many participants also agreed that recovery may not necessarily involve eliminating voices. Additionally, clients' abilities to advocate for themselves and utilize social support were identified as essential factors for successful recovery.

This study provided additional research in several areas of sparse but emerging literature, including clinicians' perspectives (including biases) on working with people who hear voices; healthy voice-hearers; critical theory; and positive psychology interventions for people who hear voices. Additionally, gaining perspectives from clinicians from both clinical and counseling psychology backgrounds provided richer knowledge on some of the key experiences from both types of training. Finally, with the implications provided here, readers who are interested in conducting further research, enhancing their clinical work, improving training programs, or advocating for people who experience voices, can make a difference across multiple areas.

REFERENCES

Academics for Black Survival and Wellness (2021). *Academics for Black survival and wellness anti-racism training.* Academics for Black Survival and Wellness. https://www.academics4blacklives.com/anti-racism-training

Ahn, W., Proctor, C. C., & Flanagan, E. H. (2009). Mental health clinicians' beliefs about the biological, psychological, and environmental bases of mental disorders. *Cognitive Science, 33*(2), 147-182. https://doi.org/10.111/j.1551-6709.2009.01008.x

Allport, G. W. (1954). The nature of prejudice. Addison-Wesley.

American Psychiatric Association (2000). *Diagnostic and statistical manual of mental disorders (4th ed., Text Revision).* American Psychiatric Publishing, Inc.

American Psychiatric Association. (2013). *Diagnostic and statistical manual of mental disorders* (5th ed.). American Psychiatric Publishing, Inc.

American Psychological Association. 2017. *Multicultural Guidelines: An Ecological Approach to Context, Identity, and Intersectionality.* Retrieved from: http://www.apa.org/about/policy/multicultural-guidelines.pdf

American Psychological Association. (2016). *2015 survey of psychology health service providers.* Washington, D.C.: Author.

Aspers, P. (2004, November). *Empirical phenomenology: An approach for qualitative research.* Paper presented to the Methodology Institute at the London School of Economics and Political Science, London, UK.

Aust, J., & Bradshaw, T. (2017). Mindfulness interventions for psychosis: A systematic

review of the literature. *Journal of Psychiatric and Mental Health Nursing, 24*(1), 69-83.

https://doi.org/10.1111/jpm.12357

Baumeister, D., Sedgwick, O., Howes, O., & Peters, E. (2017). Auditory verbal

hallucinations and continuum models of psychosis: A systematic review of the

healthy voice-hearer literature. *Clinical Psychology Review, 51*, 125-141.

https://doi.org/10.1016/j.cpr.2016.10.010

Beck, A.T., Steer, R.A., & Brown, G.K. (1996). *Manual for the Beck Depression

Inventory-II.* Psychological Corporation.

Birchwood, M., & Macmillan, F. (1993). Early intervention in schizophrenia. *The

Australian and New Zealand Journal of Psychiatry, 27*(3), 374-378.

https://doi.org/10.3109/00048679309075792

Bolier, L., Haverman, M., Westerhof, G.J., Riper, H., Smit, F., & Bohlmeijer, E. (2013).

Positive psychology interventions: A meta-analysis of randomized controlled

studies. *BMC Public Health, 13*(119). https://doi.org/10.1186/1471-2458-13-119.

Boydell, K. M., Volpe, T., Gladstone, B. M., Stasiulis, E., & Addington, J. (2013). Youth

at ultra high risk for psychosis: Using the Revised Network Episode Model to

examine pathways to mental health care. *Early Intervention in Psychiatry, 7*(2),

170-186. https://doi.org/10.1111/j.1751-7893.2012.00350.x

Braehler, C., Gumley, A., Harper, J., Wallace, S. Norrie, J., & Gilbert, P. (2013).

Exploring changes processes in compassion focused therapy in psychosis: Results

of a feasibility randomized controlled trial. *The British Journal of Clinical

Psychology, 52*(2), 199-214. https://doi.org/10.1111/bjc.12009

Braun, V., & Clarke, V. (2013). *Successful qualitative research: A practical guide for beginners.* SAGE Publications.

Carter, L., Read, J., Pyle, M., Law, H., & Morrison, A. P. (2017). Mental health clinicians' beliefs about the causes of psychosis: Differences between professions and relationship to treatment preferences. *International Journal of Social Psychiatry, 63*(5), 426-432. https://doi.org/10.1177/0020764017709849

Castel, R. Castel, F., & Lovell, A. (1982). *The psychiatric society.* Columbia University Press.

Castelein, S., Bruggeman, R., Van Busschbach, J. T., Van Der Gaag, M., Stant, A., Knegtering, H., Wiersma, D. (2008). The effectiveness of peer support groups in psychosis: A randomized controlled trial. *Acta Psychiatrica Scandinavica, 118*(1), 64-72. https://doi.org/10.1111/j.1600-0447.2008.01216.x

Chadwick, P., Lees, S., & Birchwood, M. (1995). The omnipotence of voices. II: The Beliefs about Voices Questionnaire (BAVQ-R). *British Journal of Psychiatry,* 177, 229-232. https://doi.org/10.1016/j.psychres.2017.09.089

Chadwick, P., Hughes, S., Russell, D., Russell, I., & Dagnan, D. (2009). Mindfulness groups for distressing voices and paranoia: A replication and randomized feasibility trial. *Behavioural and Cognitive Psychotherapy, 37*(4), 403-412. https://doi.org/10.1017/S1352465809990166

Chambless, D. L., & Hollon, S. D. (1998). Defining empirically supported therapies. *Journal of Consulting and Clinical Psychology, 66*(1), 7-18. https://doi.org/10.1037//0022-006x.66.1.7

Chien, W. T., Clifton, A. V., Zhao, S., & Lui, S. (2019). Peer support for people with schizophrenia or other serious mental illness. *Cochrane Database of Systematic Reviews, 2019*(4). https://doi.org/10.1002/14651858.CD010880.pub2

Chien, W. T., Lee, I. Y. (2013). The mindfulness-based psychoeducation program for Chinese patients with schizophrenia. *Psychiatric Services, 64*(4), 376-379. https://doi.org/10.1176/appi.ps.002092012

Cook, J. A., Steigman, P., Pickett, S., Diehl, S., Fox, A., Shipley, P., et al. (2012). Randomized controlled trial of peer-led recovery education using building recovery of individual dreams and goals through education and support (BRIDGES). *Schizophrenia Research, 136*(1-3), 36-42. https://doi.org/10.1016/j.schres.2011.10.016

Council of Specialties in Professional Psychology (2019). *Specialties represented on CoS.* https://www.cospp.org/clinical-psychology

Crenshaw, K., Gotanda, N., Peller, G., & Thomas, K. (1995). *Critical race theory: The key writings that formed the movement.*

Crespo-Facorro, B., Perez-Iglesias, R., Ramirez-Bonilla, M., Martinez-Garcia, O., Llorca, J., Vazquez-Barquero, J. L. (2006). A practical clinical trial comparing haloperidol, risperidone, and olanzapine for the acute treatment of first-episode nonaffective psychosis. *Journal of Clinical Psychiatry, 2006*(67), 1511-1521. https://doi.org/10.4088/jcp.v67n1004

Creswell, J. W. (2013). *Qualitative inquiry and research design: Choosing among five approaches* (3rd ed.). Sage Publications, Inc.

Daalman, K., van Zandvoort, M., Bootsman, F., Boks, M., Kahn, R., & Sommer, I.

(2011). Auditory verbal hallucinations and cognitive functioning in healthy

individuals. *Schizophrenia Research, 132*(2-3), 203-207.

https://doi.org/10.1016/j.schres.2011.07.013

Daalman, K., Boks, M. P. M., Diederen, K. M. J., De Weijer, A. D., Blom, J. D., Kahn,

R. S., & Sommer, I. E. C. (2011). The same or different? A phenomenological

comparison of auditory verbal hallucination in healthy and psychotic individuals.

Journal of Clinical Psychiatry, 72(3), 320-325.

https://doi.org/10.4088/JCP.09m05797yel

Davies, M. F., Griffin, M., & Vice, S. (2001). Affective reactions to auditory

hallucinations in psychotic, evangelical and control groups. *The British

Journal of Clinical Psychology/the   British Psychological Society, 40*(Pt 4), 361-

370. https://doi.org/10.1348/014466501163850

Davis, L. W., Lysaker, P. H., Kristeller, J. L., Salyers, M. P., Kovach, A. C., & Woller, S.

(2015). Effect of mindfulness on vocational rehabilitation outcomes in stable

phase schizophrenia. *Psychological Services, 12*(3), 303-312. https://doi.org/

10.1037/ser0000028

Delgado-Romero, E. A., Lau, M. Y., & Shullman, S. L. (2012). *The Society of

Counseling Psychology: Historical values, themes, and patterns viewed from

the American Psychological Association presidential podium.* In N. A. Fouad, J.

A. Carter, & L. M. Subich (Eds.), *APA handbooks in psychology. APA handbook

of Counseling psychology, Vol. 1. Theories, research, and methods* (pp. 3-29).

American Psychological Association.

Dennis, C. L. (2003). Peer support within a health care context: A concept analysis. *International Journal of Nursing Studies, 2003*(40), 321-332. https://doi.org/10.1016/s0020-7489(02)00092-5

Denzin, N. K., & Lincoln, Y. S. (2018). *The SAGE handbook of qualitative research.* 5th edition. SAGE Publications.

Diener, E., Emmons, R. A., Larsen, R. J., & Griffin, S. (1985). The Satisfaction With Life Scale. *Journal of Personality Assessment, 49*(1), 71-75. https://doi.org/10.1207/s15327752jpa4901_13

Dilks, S., Tasker, F., & Wren, B. (2013). Conceptualizing the therapist's role in therapy in psychosis. *Psychology and Psychotherapy: Theory, Research, and Practice, 2013*(86), 315-333. https://doi.org/10.111/j.2044-8341.2011.02061.x

Gaertner, S.L., & Dovidio, J.F. (1986). The aversive form of racism. In J.F. Dovidio & S.L. Gaertner (Eds.), *Prejudice, discrimination, and racism* (pp. 61-89). Academic Press.

Drvaric, L., Gerritsen, C., Rashid, T., Bagby, R.M., & Mizrahi, R. (2015). High stress, low resilience in people at clinical high risk for psychosis: Should we consider a strengths-based approach? *Canadian Psychology, 56*(3), 332-347. https://doi.org/10.1037/cap0000035

Eisen, S. V., Schultz, M. R., Mueller, L. N., Degenhart, C., Clark, J. A., Resnick, S. G., et al. (2012). Outcome of a randomized study of a mental health peer education and support group in the VA. *Psychiatric Services, 63*(12), 1243-1246. https://doi.org/10.1176/appi.ps.201100348

Elkins, D. N. (2009). The medical model in psychotherapy: Its limitations and failures.

    Journal of Humanistic Psychology, 49(1), 66-84.

    https://doi.org/10.1177/0022167807307901

Emsley, R. A. (1999). Risperidone in the treatment of first-episode psychotic patients:

    double-blind multicenter study. *Schizophrenia Bulletin, 1999*(25), 721-729.

    https://doi.org/10.1093/oxforjournals.schbul.a033413

Fava, G. A., & Tomba, E. (2009). Increasing psychological well-being and resilience by

    psychotherapeutic methods. *Journal of Personality, 77*(6), 1903-1934.

    https://doi.org/ 10.1111/j.1467-6494.2009.00604.x

Ferrari, M., Flora, N., Anderson, K. K., Tuck, A., Archie, S., Kidd, S., & McKenzie, K.

    (2015). The African, Caribbean and European (ACE) Pathways to Care study: A

    qualitative exploration of similarities and differences between African-origin,

    Caribbean-origin and European-origin groups in pathways to care for psychosis.

    BMJ Open 5. https://doi.org/10.1136/bmjopen-2014-006562

Fischer, C. T. & Wertz, F. J. (1979). *Empirical phenomenological analyses of being*

    criminally victimized. In A. Giorgi, R. Knowles, & D. L. Smith (Eds.).

Galderisi, S., Farden, A., & Kaiser, S. (2017). Dissecting negative symptoms of

    schizophrenia: History, assessment, pathophysiological mechanisms and

    treatment. *Schizophrenia Research, 186*(1-2).

    https://doi.org/10.1016/j.schres.2016.04.046

Gelso, C., & Fretz, B. (2001). *Counseling psychology* (2nd ed.). Thomson Wadsworth.

Girgis, R. R., Phillips, M. R., Li, X., Li, K., Jiang, H., Wu, C., Duan, N., Niu, Y.,

    Lieberman, J. A. (2018). Clozapine v. chlorpromazine in treatment-naïve, first-episode schizophrenia: 9-year outcomes of a randomized clinical trial. *The British Journal of Psychiatry, 199*(4), 281-288.

https://doi.org/10.1192/bjp.bp.110.081471

Glaser, B. G., & Strauss, A. L. (1967). *The discovery of grounded theory: Strategies for qualitative research.*

Goffman, E. (1963). *Stigma: Notes on the management of spoiled identity*. Prentice-Hall.

Greenwald, A. G., McGhee, D. E., & Schwartz, J. L. K. (1998). Measuring individual differences in implicit cognition: The implicit association test. *Journal of Personality and Social Psychology, 74*(6), 1464-1480.

https://doi.org/10.1037/0022-3514.74.6.1464

Gronholm, P. C., Thornicroft, G., Laurens, K. R., & Evans-Lacko, S. (2017). Mental health- related stigma and pathways to care for people at risk of psychotic disorders or experiencing first-episode psychosis: A systematic review. *Psychological Medicine, 2017*(47), 1867-1879.

https://doi.org/10.1017/S0033291717000344

Haddock, G., McCarron, J., Tarrier, N., & Faragher, E. B. (1999). Scales to measure dimensions of hallucinations and delusions: The psychotic symptom rating scales (PSYRATS). *Psychological Medicine, 29*(4), 879-889.

https://doi.org/10.1017/s0033291799008661

Hansson, L., Jormfeldt, H., Svedberg, P., & Svensson, B. (2013). *International Journal of Social Psychiatry, 59*(1), 48-54. https://doi.org/10.1177/0020764011423176

Hays, D. G., & Singh, A. A. (2012). *Qualitative inquiry in clinical and educational settings*. The Guilford Press.

Hayward, M., Denney, J., Vaughan, S., & Fowler, D. (2008). The voice and you:

    Development and psychometric evaluation of a measure of relationships with

    voices. *Clinical Psychology & Psychotherapy, 15*(1), 1-59.

    https://doi.org/10.1002/cpp.561

Honig, A., Romme, M. A., Ensink, B. J., Escher, S. D., Pennings, M. H., & deVries, M.

    W. (1998). Auditory hallucinations: A comparison between patients and n

    nonpatients. *The Journal of Nervous and Mental Disease, 186*(10), 646-651.

    https://doi.org/10.1097/000503-19981000-0009

Husserl, E. (1970). *The crisis of European sciences and transcendental phenomenology*

    (D. Carr, Trans.). Northwestern University Press.

Jacob, K. S. (2015). Recovery model of mental illness: A complementary approach to

    psychiatric care. *Indian Journal of Psychological Medicine, 37*(2), 117-119.

    https://doi.org/10.4103/0253-7176.155605

Jackson-Best, F., & Edwards, N. (2018). Stigma and intersectionality: A systematic

    review of systematic reviews across HIV/AIDS, mental illness, and physical

    disability. *BMC Public Health* (2018). https://doi.org/10.1186/s12899-018-5861-3

Jones, N., Rosen, C., Helm, S., O'Neill, S., Davidson, L., & Shattell, M. (2019).

    Psychosis in public mental health: Provider perspectives on clinical

    relationships and barriers to the improvement of services. *American Journal*

    of Orthopsychiatry, 89(1), 95-103. https://doi.org/10.1037/ort0000341

Kabisch, M., Ruckes, C., Seibert-Grafe, M. K., & Blettner, M. (2011). Randomized

    controlled trials: Part 17 of a series on evaluation of scientific publications.

Deutsches Arzteblatt International, 108(39): 663-668.

https://doi.org/10.3238/arztebl.2011.0663

Kay, S. R., Fiszbein, A., & Opler, L. A. (1987). The positive and negative syndrome

scale (PANSS) for schizophrenia. *Schizophrenia Bulletin, 13*(2), 261-276.

https://doi.org/10.1093/schbul/13.2.261

Kennedy, L., & Xyrichis, A. (2017). Cognitive behavioral therapy compared with non-

specialized therapy for alleviating the effect of auditory hallucinations in people

with reoccurring schizophrenia: A systematic review and meta-analysis.

Community Mental Health Journal, 53, 127-133.

https://doi.org/10.1007/s10597-016-0030-6

Khoury, B., Lecomte, T., Fortin, G., Masse, M., Therien, P., Bouchard, V., Chapleau,

M.A., Paguin, K., & Hoffman, S.G. (2013). Mindfulness-based therapy: A

comprehensive meta-analysis. *Clinical Psychology Review, 33*(6), 763-771.

https://doi.org/10.1016/j.cpr.2013.05.005

Kidd, S. A., George, L., O'Connell, M., Sylvestre, J., Kirkpatrick, H., Browne, G.,

Odueyungbo, A. O., & Davidson, L. (2011). Recovery-oriented service provision

and clinical outcomes in assertive community treatment. *Psychiatric*

Rehabilitation Journal, 34(3), 194-201.

https://doi.org/10.2975/34.3.2011.194.201

Kravik, B., Laroi, F., Kalhovde, A. M., Hugdahl, K., Kompus, K., Salvesen, O. ... Vedul

Kjelsas, E. (2015). Prevalence of auditory verbal hallucination in a general

population: A group comparison study. *Scandinavian Journal of Psychology,*

56(5), 508-515. https://doi.org/10.111/sjop.12236

Lamb, J., Bower, P., Rogers, A., Dowrick, C., & Gask, L. (2011). Access to mental

health in primary care: A qualitative meta-synthesis of evidence from the

experience of people from "hard to reach" groups. *Health, 16*(1), 76-104.

https://doi.org/10.1177/1363459311403945

Langer, A. I., Cangas, A. J., Salcedo, E., & Fuentes, B. (2012). Applying mindfulness

therapy in a group of psychotic individuals: A controlled study. *Behavioural and

Cognitive Psychotherapy, 40*(1), 105-109.

https://doi.org/10.1017/S1352465811000464

Larsson, P., Brooks, O., & Loewenthal, D. (2012). Counselling psychology and

diagnostic categories: A critical literature review. *Counselling Psychology

Review, 27*(3), 55-67. https://doi.org/10.5348/P13-2017-10-RA-1

Lehman, A. F., Lieberman, J. A., Dixon, L.B., McGlashan, A. L., Perkins, D. O., &

Kreyenbuhl, J. (2010). *Practice guideline for the treatment of patients with

schizophrenia* (2nd ed.).

Leucht, S., Tardy, M., Komossa, K., Heres, S., Kissling, M. D., Salanti, G., Davis, J. M.

(2012). Antipsychotic drugs versus placebo for relapse prevention in

schizophrenia: A systematic review and meta-analysis. *The Lancet, 379*(9381),

2063-2071. https://doi.org/10.1016/S0140-6736(12)60239-6

Li, M., Santpere, G., Kawasawa, Y. I., Evgrafov, O. V., Gulden, F. O., Pochareddy, S.,

Sestan, N. (2018). Integrative functional genomic analysis of human brain

development neuropsychiatric risks. *Science, 362*(6420).

https://doi.org/10.1126/science.aat7615

Li, J., Fan, Y., Zhong, H. Q., Duan, X. L., Chen, W., Evans-Lacko, S., & Thornicroft, G. (2019). Effectiveness of an anti-stigma training on improving attitudes and decreasing discrimination towards people with mental disorders among care assistant workers in   Guangzhou, China. *International Journal of Mental Health Systems, 13*(1). https://doi.org/10.1186/s13033-018-0259-2

Longden, E., Madill, E., & Waterman, M.G. (2012). Dissociation, trauma, and the role of lived experience: Toward a new conceptualization of voice hearing. *Psychological Bulletin, 138*(1), 28-76. https://doi.org/10.1037/a0025995

Lopez, S. J., Magyar-Moe, J. L., Petersen, S. E., Ryder, J. A., Krieshok, T. S., Koetting-O'Byrne, K., Lichtenberg, J. W., & Fry, N. A. (2006). Counseling psychology's focus on positive aspects of human functioning. *The Counseling Psychologist, 34*(2), 205-227. https://doi.org/10.1177/0011000005283393

Lopez-Navarro, E., Del Canto, C., Belber, M., Mayol, A., Fernandez-Alonso, O., Lluis, J., Munar, E., Chadwick, P. (2015). Mindfulness improves psychological quality of life in community-based patients with severe mental health problems: A pilot randomized clinical trial. *Schizophrenia Research, 168* (1-2), 530-536. https://doi.org/10.1016/j.schres.2015.08.016

Lund, N. (2009). Document theory. *Annual Review of Information Science and Technology, 43*(1), 1-55. https://doi.org/10.1002/aris.2009.1440430116

Lyubomirski, S., Sousa, L., & Dickerhoof, R. (2006). The costs and benefits of writing, talking, and thinking about life's triumphs and defeats. *Journal of Personality and Social Psychology, 90*(4), 692-708. https://doi.org/10.1037/0022-3 3514.90.4.692

Mahlke, C. I., Priebe, S., Heumann, K., Daubmann, A., Wegscheider, K., Bock, T. (2017). Effectiveness of one-to-one peer support for patients with severe m mental illness – A randomized controlled trial. *European Psychiatry, 2017*(42), 103-110. https://doi.org/10.1016/j.eurpsy.2016.12.007

Malla, A., Joober, R., & Garcia, A. (2015). "Mental illness is like any other medical illness": A critical examination of the statement and its impact on patient care and society. *Journal of Psychiatry & Neuroscience, 40*(3), 147-150. https://doi.org/10.1503/jpn.150099

Martinussen, M. (2018). Critical social psychology and interdisciplinary studies of personal life: Greater than the sum of its parts. *Social and Personality Psychology Compass, 13*(1). https://doi.org/10.111/spc3.12428

Maslow, A. H. (1970). *Motivation and Personality* (2nd ed.). Harper & Row.

May, S. (1997). Critical ethnography. In Hornberger, N. H., & Corson, P. (Eds.), *Encyclopedia of Language and Education: Research Methods in Language and Education* (pp. 197-206). Springer.

McGoury, P. D., & Yung, A. R. (1996). The initial prodrome in psychosis: Descriptive and qualitative aspects. *The Australian and New Zealand Journal of Psychiatry, 30*(5), 587-599. https://doi.org/10.3109/00048679609062654

Menon, M., Balzan, R. P., Harper, K., Kumar, D., Andersen, D., Moritz, S., & Woodward, T. (2017). Psychosocial approaches in the treatment of psychosis: Cognitive behavior therapy for psychosis (CBT for psychosis) and metacognitive training (MCT). *Clinical Schizophrenia & Related Psychoses, 11*(3), 157-1 163. https://doi.org/10.3371/CSRP.MEBA.022015

Meyer, P. S., Johnson, D. P., Parks, A., Iwanski, C., & Penn, D. L. (2012). Positive

living: A pilot study of group positive psychotherapy for people with

schizophrenia. *The Journal of Positive Psychology, 7*(3), 239-248.

https://doi.org/10.1080/17439760.2012.677467

Miller, S. D., Duncan, B. L., Brown, J., Sparks, J. A., & Claud, D. A. (2003). The

Outcome Rating Scale: A preliminary study of the reliability, validity, and

feasibility of a brief visual analog measure. *Journal of Brief Therapy, 2*(2), 91-

100.

Moran, D., (2013). *Edmund Husserl and phenomenology. Philosophy of Mind: The Key

Thinkers.* Bloomsbury.

Moritz, S., Thoering, T., Kuhn, S., Willenborg, B., Westermann, S., & Nagel, M. (2015).

Metacognition-augmented cognitive remediation training reduces jumping to

conclusions and overconfidence but not neurocognitive deficits in psychosis.

Frontiers in Psychology, 6(1048), 1-11. https://doi.org/10.3389/fpsyg.2015.01048

National Hearing Voices Network (2021). *Hearing Voices Network: For people who hear

voices, see visions or have other unusual perceptions.* Hearing Voices Network.

https://www.hearing-voices.org.

Newton-Howes, G., & Wood, R. (2011). Cognitive behavioural therapy and the

psychopathology of schizophrenia: Systematic review and meta-analysis.

Psychology and Psychotherapy: Theory, Research and Practice, 2013(86), 127-

138. https://doi.org/10.111/j.2044-8341.2011.02048.x

Paterson, C., Karatzias, T., Dickson, A., Harper, S., Dougall, N., & Hutton, P. (2018).

Psychological therapy for inpatients receiving acute mental health care: A systematic review and meta-analysis of controlled trials. *British Journal of C*

Clinical Psychology, 57(4), 453-472. https://doi.org/10.1111/bjc.12182

Penn, D. L., Meyer, P. S., Evans, E., Wirth, R. J., Cai, K., & Burchinal, M. (2009). A

randomized controlled trial of group cognitive-behavioral therapy vs. enhanced

supportive therapy for auditory hallucinations. *Schizophrenia Research, 109*(1-3),

52-59. https://doi.org/10.1016/j.schres.2008.12.009

Perrin, M. A., Kantrowitz, J. T., Silipo, G., Dias, E., Jabado, O., & Javitt, D. C. (2018).

Mismatch negativity (MMN) to spatial deviants and behavioral spatial

discrimination ability in the etiology of auditory verbal hallucinations and

thought disorder in schizophrenia. *Schizophrenia Research*, 191, 140-147.

https://doi.org/10.1016/j.schres.2017.05.012

Pluye, P., Robert, E., Cargo, M., Bartlett, G., O'Cathain, A., Griffiths, F., Boardman, F.,

Gagnon, M.P., & Rousseau, M.C. (2011). Proposal: A mixed methods appraisal

tool for systematic mixed studies reviews.

http://mixedmethodsappraisaltoolpublic.pbworks.com

Ralph, R. O. (2000). Recovery. *Psychiatric Rehabilitation Skills, 4*(3), 480-517.

https://doi.org/10.1080/10973430008408634

Randal, P., Lampshire, D., Symes, J., & Hamer, H. (2009). "The Re-covery Model" – An

integrative developmental stress-vulnerability-strengths approach to mental

health. (Psychosis) *Psychological, Social, and Integrative Approaches, 1*(1-12).

https://doi.org/10.1080/1752243092948167

Rashid, T., & Ostermann, R.F. (2009) Strength-based assessment in clinical practice. *Journal of Clinical Psychology: In Session, 65*(5), 488-498. https://doi.org/10.1002/jclp.20595

Reeves, S., Albert, M., Kuper, A., & Hodges, B. D. (2008). Qualitative research – Why use theories in qualitative research? *British Medical Journal, 337*(7670), 631-634. https://doi.org/10.1136/bmj.a949

Roe, D., & Davidson, L. (2005). Self and narrative in schizophrenia: Time to author a new story. *Medical Humanities, 31*(2), 89-94. https://doi.org/10.1136/jmh.2005.000214

Roe, D., Yanos, P.T., & Lysaker, P.H. (2006). Coping with psychosis: An integrative developmental framework. *Journal of Nervous and Mental Disease, 194*(12), 917-924. https://doi.org/ 10.1097/01.nmd.0000249108.61185.d3

Rose, N. (1985). *The Psychological Complex: psychology, politics and society in England 1869-1939.* Routledge and Kegan Paul.

Rusch, N., Corrigan, P. W., Wassel, A., Michaels, P., Olschewski, M., Wilkniss, S., & Batia, K. (2009). A stress-coping model of mental illness stigma: Predictors of cognitive stress appraisal. *Schizophrenia Research, 110*(1-3), 59-64. https://doi.org/10.1016/j.schres.2009.01.006

Rusch, N., Heekeren, K., Theodoridou, A., Dvorsky, D., Muller, M., Paust, T., Corrigan, P. W., Walitza, S., & Rossler, W. (2013). Attitudes towards help-seeking and stigma among young people at risk for psychosis. *Psychiatry Research* (2013). https://doi.org/10.1016/j.psychres.2013.08.028

Saayman, N. (2017). Flying blind in the psychotic storm. *Psycho-analytic Psychotherapy in South Africa, 25*(1). https://hdl.handle.net/10520/EJC-76e95f641

Saha, Bhowmik, S., Chant, D., & McGrath, J. (2008). Meta-analyses of the incidence and prevalence of schizophrenia: Conceptual and methodological issues. *International Journal of Methods in Psychiatric Research, 17*(1), 55-61. https://doi.org/10.1002/mpr.240

Savickas, M. L. (2003). Introduction to the Special Issue, *Career Development Quarterly. 52*(1), 4-7. https://doi.org/10.1002/j.2161-0045.2003.tb00621.x

Schrank, B., Riches, S., Coggins, T., Rashid, T., Tylee, A., & Slade, M. (2014). WELLFOCUS positive psychotherapy: Modified positive psychotherapy to improve well-being in psychosis: Study protocol for a pilot randomized controlled trial. *Trials, 203*(2014). https://doi.org/10.1186/1745-6215-15-203

Schultze-Lutter, Klosterkotter, J., Picker, H., Eckhard-Michael, S., & Ruhrmann, S. (2007). Predicting first-episode psychosis by basic symptom criteria. *Clinical Neuropsychiatry, 4*(1), 11-22. https://doi.org/10.2174/138161212700316064

Segal, Z. V., Williams, J. M. G., & Teasdale, J. D. (2002). Mindfulness-based cognitive therapy for depression: A new approach to preventing relapse. Guilford.

Seligman, M. E. P. & Csikszentmihalyi, M. (2000). Positive psychology: An introduction. *American Psychologist, 55*(1), 5-14. https://doi.org/10.1037/0003-066X.55.1.5

Seligman, M. E. P. (2002). Authentic Happiness: Using the new positive psychology to realize your potential for lasting fulfillment. Free Press.

Seligman, M. E. P. & Pawelski, J. O. (2003). Positive psychology: FAQs. *Psychological*

Inquiry, 14(2), 159-163. https://ww.jstor.org/stable/1449825

Seligman, M. E. P., Parks, A. C., & Steen, T. (2004). A balanced psychology and a full

life. *Philosophical Transactions B, 359*(1449),1379-1381. https://doi.org/

10.1098/rstb.2004.1513

Shawyer, F., Farhall, J., Mackinnon, A., Trauer, T., Sims, E., Ratcliff, K., ... Copolov, D.

(2012). A randomized controlled trial of acceptance-based cognitive behavioural

therapy for command hallucinations in psychotic disorders. *Behaviour Research*

and Therapy, 50(2), 110-121. https://doi.org/10.1016/j.brat.2011.11.007

Sherbourne, C. D., Allen, H. M., Kamberg, C. J., & Wells, K. B. (1992). Physical

psychophysiologic symptoms measure. In A. L. Steward & J. E. Ware (Eds.),

Measuring functioning and well-being (pp. 260-272). Duke University Press.

Shonin, E., Van Gordon, W., & Griffiths, M. D. (2014). Are there risks associated with

using mindfulness for the treatment of psychopathology? *Clinical Practice,*

15(1), 389-392. https://doi.org/10.1146/annurev-clinpsy-021815-093423

Siddaway, A. P., Wood, A. M., Taylor, P. J. (2017). The Center for Epidemiologic

Studies-Depression (CES-D) scale measures a continuum from well-being to

depression: Testing   two key predictions of positive clinical psychology.

Journal of Affective Disorders, 213, 180-186.

https://doi.org/10.1016/j.jad2017.02.015

Slade, M. (2010). Mental illness and well-being: The central importance of positive

psychology and recovery approaches. *BMC Health Services Research, 10*(26).

Smith, J. A., & Osborn, M. (2003). Interpretative Phenomenological Analysis. In J. A.

Smith (Ed.), Qualitative Psychology: A Practical Guide to Methods (pp. 53-80).

Sage.

Sommer, I. E., Derwort, M. C., Daalman, K., de Weijer, A. D., Liddle, P. F., & Boks, M.

P. M. (2010). Healthy individuals with auditory verbal hallucination: Who are

they? Psychiatric assessments of a selected sample of 103 subjects. *Schizophrenia*

Bulletin, 36(3), 633-641. https://doi.org/10.1093/schbul/sbn130

Sorrell, E., Hayward, M., & Meddings, S. (2010). Interpersonal processes and hearing

voices: A study of the association between relating to voices and distress in

clinical and non-clinical hearers. *Behavioural and Cognitive Psychotherapy,*

38(2), 127-140. https://doi.org/10.1017/S1352465809990506

Steinberg, J., & White, R. (1996). The advantages of the disease model. *Journal of the*

Maryland State Dental Association, 39(2), 87-88.

Stewart, A. L., Hays, R. D., & Ware, J. E. (1988). The MOS short-form general health

survey: Reliability and validity in a patient population. *Medical Care, 26*(7),

724-735. https://doi.org/10.1097/00005650-198807000-00007

Stull, L. G., McGrew, J. H., Salyers, M. P., & Ashburn-Nardo, L. (2013). Implicit and

explicit stigma of mental illness: Attitudes in an evidence-based practice.

Journal of Nervous and Mental Disease, 201(12), 1072-1079.

https://doi.org/10.1097/NMD.0000000000000056

Switaj, P., Anczewska, M., Chrostek, A., Sabariego, C., Cieza, A., Bickenbach, J., &

Chatterji, S. (2012). Disability and schizophrenia: A systematic review of experienced psychosocial difficulties. *BMC Psychiatry,* 12, *193(*2012).

https://doi.org/10.1186/1471- 244X-12-193.

Taylor, G., & Murray, C. (2012). A qualitative investigation into non-clinical voice

hearing: What factors may protect against distress? *Mental Health Religion &*

Culture, 15(4), 373-388. https://doi.org/10.1080/13674676.2011.577411

Thomas, P., & Longden, E. (2015). Phenomenology in a different key: Narrative,

meaning and madness. *Philosophy, Psychiatry, & Psychology, 22*(3), 187-192.

https://doi.org/10.1353/ppp.2015.0031

Trace, C. B. (2016). Phenomenology, experience, and the essence of documents as

objects. *Proceedings of the Ninth International Conference of Conceptions of*

Library and Information Science, Uppsala, Sweden, June 27-29, 2016.

van Os, J., Linscott, R.J., Myin-Germeys, I., Delespaul, P., & Krabbendam, L. (2008). A

systematic review and meta-analysis of the psychosis continuum: Evidence for a

psychosis proneness-persistence-impairment model of psychotic disorder.

Psychological Medicine, 39(2), 179-195.

https://doi.org/10.1017/S0033291708003814

Vanstone, M., Rewegan, A., Brundisini, F., Giacomini, M., Kandasamy, S., & DeJean, D.

2017). Diet modification challenges faced by marginalized and nonmarginalized

adults with type 2 diabetes: A systematic review and qualitative meta-synthesis.

Chronic Illness, 13(3), 217-235. https://doi.org/10.1177/1742395316675024

Walsh, F. (2004). Family resilience: A framework for clinical practice. (2004). *Family*

Process, 42(1), 1-18. https://doi.org/10.111/j.1545-5300.2003.00001.x

Wampold, B.E. & Imel Z.E. (2015). *The great psychotherapy debate: The evidence for what makes psychotherapy work* (2nd edition). Routledge.

Watson, D., Clark, L. A., & Tellegen, A. (1988). Development and validation of brief measures of positive and negative affect: The PANAS scales. *Journal of Personality and Social Psychology, 54*(6), 1063-1070. https://doi.org/10.1037/0022-3514.54.6.1063

Whiteley, J. M. (1984). Editor's Introduction. *The Counseling Psychologist, 12*(2). https://doi.org/10.1177/001100006900100301

Wood, A. M., & Johnson, J. (2016). The Wiley Handbook of Positive Clinical Psychology: An Integrative Approach to Studying and Improving Well-Being. Blackwell Publishing.

Wood, A. M., & Tarrier, N. (2010) Positive clinical psychology: A new vision and strategy for integrated research and practice. *Clinical Psychology Review, 30*(7), 819-829. https://doi.org/10.1016/j.cpr.2010.06.003

Woods, A., Jones, N., Alderson-Day, B., Callard, F., & Fernyhough, C. (2015). Experiences of hearing voices: Analysis of a novel phenomenological survey. *The Lancet Psychiatry, 2*(4), 323-331. H https://doi.org/10.1016/S2215-0366(15)0006-1

Xu, Z., Muller, M., Heekeren, K., Theodoridou, A., Dvorsky, D. N., Metzler, S., … Rusch, N. 2016). Self-labelling and stigma as predictors of attitudes towards help-seeking among people at risk of psychosis: 1-year follow-up. *European Archives of Psychiatry and Clinical Neuroscience, 266(*1). https://10.1007/s00406-015-0576-2

Yalom, I.D. (1980). *Existential psychotherapy.* Basic Books.

Yazici, E., Cilli, A. B., Baysan, H., Ince, M., Bosgelmez, S., Bilgic, S., Aslan, B., & Erol, A. (2017). Antipsychotic use pattern in schizophrenia outpatients: Correlates of polypharmacy. *Clinical Practice and Epidemiology in Mental Health, 2017*(13), 92-103. https://10.2174/1745017901713010092

Yennari, A. (2011). *Living with schizophrenia: A phenomenological investigation.*

Yip, K.S. (2005). A strengths perspective in understanding and working with clients with psychosis and records of violence. *Journal of Humanistic Psychology, 45*(4), 446-464. https://doi.org/10.1177/0022167805280263

Zimmermann, G., Favrod, J., Trieu, V. H., & Pomini, V. (2005). The effect of cognitive behavioral treatment on the positive symptoms of schizophrenia spectrum disorders: A   meta-analysis. *Schizophrenia Research, 77*(1), 1-9. https://doi.org/10.1016/j.schres.2005.02.018